D. R. INOGAMOVA

Basic genetics and inherited disorders in child development

D. R. INOGAMOVA

Basic genetics and inherited disorders in child development

ScienciaScripts

Cover image: www.ingimage.com

This book is a translation from the original published under ISBN 978-620-7-80747-5.

Publisher:
Sciencia Scripts
is a trademark of
Dodo Books Indian Ocean Ltd. and OmniScriptum S.R.L publishing group

120 High Road, East Finchley, London, N2 9ED, United Kingdom
Str. Armeneasca 28/1, office 1, Chisinau MD-2012, Republic of Moldova, Europe
Printed at: see last page
ISBN: 978-620-8-35116-8

Contents

Genetics is the heart of biological science.
Only within the framework of genetics can the
diversity of life forms and processes be
understood as a unified whole.
***Ф**. Ayala, American geneticist, author of the*
textbook Modern Genetics.

INTRODUCTION

Genetics is a branch of biology that studies the material basis of heredity and variability, as well as regularities of inheritance and changes in traits in a number of generations of organisms. ***Heredity*** is understood as the property of organisms to repeat in a number of generations the traits, similar types of metabolism and individual development in general. In other words, heredity ensures the reproduction of a new generation in the strict forms of the original species through the transmission of hereditary information about traits and properties. ***Variability is the*** exact opposite property, thanks to it, new traits appear in the offspring. Modified hereditary information is transmitted in the subsequent generation from generation to generation.

Heredity as a property of all organisms has interested people since ancient times. Pre-scientific ideas about inherited differences between people probably existed already in ancient times. In statements usually attributed to Hippocrates, one can find the following statement: "..... Seed produces the whole body, healthy seed produces healthy parts of the body, sick seed produces sick parts of the body. Since, as a rule, a bald man gives birth to a bald man, a blue-eyed man to a blue-eyed man, and an oblique man to an oblique man, there is nothing to prevent the birth of long-headed men to long-headed men." The same views were held by Anaxagoras and Aristotle. Plato in his work "Politics" explains in detail how to choose spouses to give birth to children who will be able to become outstanding personalities both physically and morally.

The genius work of the scientist-encyclopaedist Abu Ali ibn Sina "Avicenna" (980 - 1037) *"Conon of Medical Science"* allowed him to become one of the greatest representatives of mankind for all time. *"Conon" - a* capital work, a real encyclopaedia of medical knowledge that mankind had accumulated by that time. In addition, it included a lot of previously unknown to medical science information in the field of surgery, diagnosis and hereditary diseases. Ibn Sina based on his scientific observations made an assumption that if a person is physically strong and healthy, his generation will be as strong and healthy, that some diseases are inherited from generation to generation.

But it was only in the 11th century that these phenomena began to be objectively studied. The Czech researcher Gregor Johann Mendel made a decisive contribution to understanding the mechanisms of trait inheritance.

He can be considered the founder of scientific genetics. In 1866, Mendel published the results of experiments on peas in his article "Experiments on plant hybrids", in which he showed that heredity is transmitted through germ cells *in the form of discrete factors* from one generation to another, *without mixing and dissolving.* However, the significance of his research was truly recognised when, in 1900, three scientists - G. De Fries, C. Correns and C. Cermak - simultaneously obtained similar results on different plant objects, which confirmed the correctness of H. Mendel's conclusions. The year 1900 became the year of birth of genetics as a science. The term *"genetics"* was introduced in 1906 by W.Batson.

The discovery of Mendel's laws caused a rapid development of the science of heredity and variability of organisms, which became known as genetics. In its development, genetics has passed through three stages, between which there are no clear boundaries. At each of them, certain human ideas about the structure of hereditary material and about the regularities of inheritance and changes in traits were formed.

The first stage is the era of "Classical Genetics" (1900 - 1930). During this time, Mendelism was finally established, the phenomenon of linked inheritance was discovered, the gene theory and the chromosomal theory of heredity were formulated. The development of the doctrine of phenotype and genotype and the interaction of genes was also important.

The second stage of genetics development is known as "Neoclassicism" (1930-1953), when biochemical methods and induced mutagenesis in genetic research were discovered. At this stage, undeniable evidence of the leading role of DNA in the phenomena of heredity and variability was obtained, the physical and chemical structure of the DNA molecule was determined, and the biological code was deciphered.

The third stage "Synthetic period of genetics development" (from 1953 to the present day). At present, the main attention is paid to the study of the fine structure and functions of the gene, the issues of regulation of gene activity. The mutation process is intensively studied, and methods of genetic engineering are being developed to artificially change hereditary properties in the desired direction.

Thus, the third, modern stage of genetics development opened up huge prospects for directed intervention in the phenomena of heredity and selection of plant and animal organisms, revealed the important role of genetics in medicine, in particular, in the study of patterns of hereditary diseases and physical anomalies of humans. In each decade of the 20th century, important discoveries were made in genetics. Gradually, this science occupied key positions and a leading position in fundamental biology.

The chronology of the most important discoveries in human genetics and medical genetics is given below (in Table 1).

Table 1.

Major discoveries in human genetics

Year	Scientific discovery	Researchers
1866	Corpuscular heredity. Laws of inheritance	H. Mendel
1876	Gemini method	F.Galton
1900	Discovery of mendelating polymorphic human traits (ABO blood groups)	K. Landsteiner
1902	Human biochemical variability, inborn errors of metabolism	A. Garrod
1903	The chromosome as a carrier of genes	W. Sutton and T. Boveri
1910	Localisation of human genes on a chromosome	E.Wilson
1911	The chromosomal theory of heredity	T.G. Morgan et al.
1927	Establishing the mutagenic effect of X-rays	G. Meller
1940	The concept of polymorphism	E. Ford
1947	Mobile genetic elements	Б. McClintock
1949	The discovery of sex chromatin	M. Barr and L. Bertram
1953	DNA structure	J. Watson and F. Crick.
1954	The role of infectious diseases in shaping the human gene pool	A.Ellison
1955	Enzymatic synthesis of RNA and DNA	O. Ochoa and A.Kornberg
1956	Determining the number of chromosomes in humans	J. Thio and A. Levan
1957	Determination of oligene determination amino acid sequences in a protein molecule	W. Ingram
1959	Chromosomal aberration as a cause of congenital anomaly in humans (Down syndrome)	J.Lejeune et al.
1959	Establishing the role of the Y chromosome in sex determination in humans	C. Ford and P. Jacobs
1960	Preparation of chromosome preparations from peripheral blood leukocytes	P.Moorhead
1961	Biochemical screening	R.Guthrie
1961	The discovery of the genetic code	M. Nirenberg
1962	Indiscriminate inactivation of one of the X chromosomes	E. Beitler

	in female individuals	
1966	Prenatal diagnosis of chromosomal diseases	M. Steele and V. Breg
1970	Differential staining of chromosomes	T. Kasperson, A.F. Zakharov
1970	Artificially synthesised gene	H.B. Koran
1978	Molecular genetic diagnostics	J.Kann
1983	Polymerase chain reaction method	C. Mullison
1985	DNA dactyloscopy method	A.Jeffries
1988	Uniparental dyssomia in humans	J. Spence et al.
1988	Pathological anatomy of the human genome as a new paradigm of medicine	B. Mac Cusick
1989	First successful attempts at gene therapy for hereditary and non-hereditary (tumours and infections) diseases	A.Anderson
1990	Genomic imprinting and imprinting diseases	J. Hall
1991	Diseases of expansion of tandem repeats	A.Verkerk et al.
1992	Classification of mitochondrial diseases	D. Wallace
1989	Deciphering the genomes of many organisms	
2002	Human genome sequencing	Result of international co-operation

Heredity and variability are the primary inherent properties of living organisms. They are the basis of all life manifestations. Without heredity and variability, the evolution of life on Earth would be impossible. Man is a "product" of the long evolution of living nature. All general biological regularities are reflected in his formation as a biological species *"Man of reason" (Homo sapiens)*.

In its development, human genetics was constantly "fed" from general biological concepts (evolutionary doctrine, ontogenesis), from genetic discoveries (Mendelism, chromosomal theory of heredity, informational role of DNA), from the achievements of theoretical and clinical medicine.

There is now no doubt that an organism is the result of a complex interaction between the genetic programme inherited from parents and diverse, constantly changing environmental conditions.

The genetic programme, on the one hand, being transmitted from generation to generation, ensures reproduction of typological characteristics of a human being as a representative of a biological species and inheritance of some, including pathological, features of parents. On the other hand, it creates each time (on the basis of genetic phenomena and regularities) an individual unique in its genotypic individuality.

The centuries-old experience of medicine convincingly testifies to the individual character of the course of pathology. The individual nature of the disease, manifested in the rate of disease development, intensity of the pathological process, specificity of its course, outcome of the disease, etc., is largely due to the genetic uniqueness of each person, inimitable ways of implementation of the genetic programme.

An applied branch of medical genetics is clinical genetics, which uses advances in medical genetics, human genetics, and general genetics to address clinical problems that arise in specific patients or their families.

Human genetics owes much of its success to medical genetics, a science that studies the role of heredity in human pathology, the patterns of transmission of hereditary diseases from generation to generation, and develops methods of diagnosis, treatment and prevention of all forms of hereditary pathology. In this direction, the achievements of both medicine and genetics are synthesised. This synthesis is aimed at fighting diseases and improving human health.

Genetics answers the following specific questions: what hereditary mechanisms maintain the homeostasis of the organism and determine the health of an individual; what is the significance of hereditary factors in the etiology of diseases; what is the ratio of hereditary and environmental factors in the pathogenesis of diseases; what is the role of hereditary factors in determining the clinical picture of diseases, whether hereditary constitution affects the process of recovery and the outcome of the disease; what hereditary factors determine the specificity of pharmacological and other types of treatment.

Currently, medical genetics is intensively developing in different directions: the study of the human genome, cytogenetics, molecular and biochemical genetics, immunogenetics, clinical genetics, and ecogenetics.

Through the interpenetration of ideas, concepts and methods, general genetics, human genetics and medical genetics have greatly enriched each other, ultimately contributing 7
to ensure that the achievements of science are realised in practice not only by the doctor, but also by the teacher-defectologist, psychologist and preschool education specialist.

As a result of a century of development of human genetics as a science, the main provisions of genetics have been formed, knowledge of which is obligatory for an educated teacher-defectologist, psychologist and preschool education specialist.

1. Hereditary diseases are part of the total hereditary variability in humans. There is no sharp boundary between hereditary variability leading to variations in normal traits and variability causing hereditary diseases. Both neutral and pathological mutations can occur in the same genes.

2. The development of inherited traits or diseases involves the human genotype and the external environment. In all life manifestations, there is always an interaction between heredity and environment. Although heredity (genotype) plays a determining role for the development of some traits or diseases, and the external environment plays a significant role for the development of others (by hypothermia, malnutrition, emotional or mental stress, etc.), there are no traits that depend only on heredity or only on the environment.

3. Humanity is "burdened" with a huge "load" of various mutations, the accumulation of which occurred in the process of long evolution. The constantly running mutation process supplied new mutations to the gene pool of mankind, and natural selection preserved and multiplied or led to their disappearance.

4. If a few decades ago they talked about hundreds of hereditary diseases, nowadays, when describing any diseases, including infectious diseases, we have to some extent to take into account the hereditary structure of the organism and its role in the etiology and pathogenesis of the disease. For a thinking pedagogical worker, genetic concepts can become a "guiding star" both in the practical activity of a pedagogue, diagnosis and prevention among their relatives.

5. The progress of medicine and society leads to an increase in the life expectancy of patients with hereditary diseases, restoration of their reproductive function and, consequently, to an increase in their number in the population. A sick person or a carrier of a pathological condition is a full member of society and has equal rights with a healthy person. Concepts such as eugenics, the degeneration of families with hereditary pathology, the incurability of hereditary diseases, the prohibition of marriage or sterilisation on genetic grounds are a thing of the past. In the diagnosis, treatment and prevention of hereditary diseases, modern medicine and pedagogy have great possibilities, which will become even greater in the future. The importance of genetics for pedagogy cannot be overestimated.

Firstly, as part of the theoretical foundation of medicine, genetics expands and deepens the biological thinking of a specialist. The future pedagogue through understanding the laws of heredity and variability should really represent all stages of individual human development from the angle of implementation of the programme inherited by an individual in specific environmental conditions. Genetic knowledge is necessary for new methods of diagnostics, treatment and prevention of hereditary diseases, education and understanding of such sick children.

Secondly, the achievements of medical genetics are effectively implemented in all sections of pedagogy and psychology. Hereditary diseases occupy a significant place in the work of every teacher educator due to their frequency and severity. Hereditary diseases include a wide range of diseases of various nosological classes. These are numerous diseases of internal organs, metabolism, blood, endocrine system, skin, eyes, genitourinary system, nervous and mental diseases, etc. About 5 per cent of children are born with hereditary and congenital diseases. Hereditary diseases include such widespread visual defects as myopia, hyperopia and colour blindness (it occurs in 0.5% of women and 8% of men). Diseases with hereditary predisposition include atherosclerosis, heart defects, schizophrenia, childhood autism and others. Consequently, every teacher-defectologist, psychologist and preschool education specialist may encounter hereditary pathologies in their daily work.

Thanks to the successes of medical science and scientific and technical achievements of recent years, the percentage of recognition of genetically determined pathology in the structure of morbidity, mortality and disability of the population is increasing.

For example, in countries with developed health systems, genetic factors are responsible for:

80% mental retardation;

70% congenital blindness;

50% congenital deafness;

40-50% of spontaneous abortions and miscarriages;

20-30% of infant mortality.

Among the reasons for hospitalisation of children in non-specialised hospitals, hereditary diseases account for 20 to 40% of all cases. In other words, on average, every fourth child admitted to a general hospital is a child with a hereditary pathology. Naturally, among children with mental retardation, hearing loss, deafness and loss of sight, the number of patients with hereditary diseases is much higher.

Hereditary pathology can "haunt" a person at all stages of life: from birth to old age. Consequently, not only medical, but also pedagogical assistance and psychological support should be provided not only to the sick child, but also to his/her family. In this extremely important case, the role of the educator is invaluable.

Hereditary diseases had long been untreatable, and the only method of prevention was the recommendation to abstain from childbearing.

Modern medical genetics is equipped with methods of early pre-symptomatic and even prenatal diagnosis of hereditary diseases. Methods of preimplantation diagnostics are being intensively developed.

The development of genetics, which has achieved unprecedented success in recent years, predetermines the birth of a new approach to understanding not only medical, but also psychological, pedagogical and other problems related to the human factor. The preliminary results of twin and family studies aimed at studying the contribution of genetic factors to the formation of temperament properties and some personality traits are now confirmed by the results of molecular genetic studies. Studies of the genetic control of some neurotransmitter systems of the brain have made it possible to discover and identify genetic systems that form the basis and mechanisms of memory, contributing to the development of addictive or aggressive behaviour.

It is obvious that the formation of adequate behaviour in a child (both normal and abnormal), the development of certain skills, adaptation and learning processes should be carried out on the basis of understanding the causes, structure of defects and the nature of their interaction with other systems of the body. Understanding the problems of the emergence and formation of abnormality in a child is a prerequisite for successful and qualified pedagogical intervention.

Knowledge of the laws of heredity plays a huge role in pedagogical education. All human behaviour is to a greater or lesser extent linked to phylogenetic inheritance. To understand the subtle mechanisms of this relationship requires not superficial but profound knowledge.

The methodological role of genetics in education predetermines special requirements for its teaching, which should combine breadth of coverage, scientific depth and accessibility of presentation. This textbook deals at an appropriate level with all sections of the modern science of genetics necessary for understanding human genetics and behaviour, so it is hoped that it will be useful to all students and researchers studying these areas.

Brief but coherent presentations of the basic tenets of genetics are especially needed in pre-school departments.

Together with a doctor, a pedagogical defectologist, a psychologist and a preschool education specialist can actively participate in putting medical genetics into practice for the sake of a happy family with healthy offspring.

Control Questions:

1. What is the essence of the phenomena of heredity and variability?
2. What is genetics, history of development of genetics?
3. What does medical genetics study?
4. What are the basic statements of genetics of which knowledge is essential for an educated teacher?
5. Provide key examples of the importance of medical genetics in pedagogy.

CHAPTER I

THE CYTOLOGICAL BASIS OF HEREDITY.

1.1. CELL STRUCTURE AND FUNCTIONS

All living organisms, with the exception of viruses, consist of cells. Cells, most often represented by microscopic formations, possess all the most important vital properties: self-regulation, self-reproduction, unity of structure and function, historical development, etc. Cells are constantly undergoing processes of metabolism and energy transformation.

The science that studies the structure and functioning of cells is called *cytology* (from Greek *kytos* - cell + *logos* - science). The development and establishment of cytology was largely determined by the improvement of microscopic techniques, as cells are difficult to study with the naked eye.

In 1665, the English naturalist R. Hooke first reported the existence of cells. He examined thin slices of cork under his improved microscope and found small empty pores and cells, which he called cells. Strictly speaking, in a slice of cork R. Hooke observed dead cell walls, deprived of the living content that filled them. Examining under the microscope various parts of other plants, in particular carrots, burdock, fern, he found the same plan of structure as that of cork.

In 1677, M. Malpighi reported on the cellular structure of all the plants he had studied. The prominent scientist of the XVII century Anthony van Leeuwenhoek, examining a drop of water under a microscope, discovered the simplest unicellular organisms. For a long time, the main structural component of a cell was recognised as its membrane.

After technical improvements in the quality of lenses in the early 19th century, attention to microscope research increased rapidly. In 1825, the Czech scientist J. Purkinje showed that inside the cell there is a gelatinous substance, later called cytoplasm. The English botanist R. Brown described the nucleus of the cell. The German botanist M. Schleiden in 1837 concluded that all plant cells contain nuclei.

In 1839, the German zoologist T. Schwann, summarising his own experimental data and the results of other scientists, formulated the concept now known as the *cell theory*.

According to cellular theory:

1) the cell is the basic element of life;

2) Any organisms are made up of one or many cells.
Indeed, despite the enormous diversity of living beings, differing in size, shape, habitat, mode of movement, energy supply, etc., the basis of their morphofunctional organisation is cells. R.Virchow in 1855 added to these two postulates a fundamental position: *"Omnis cellula e cellulae" - "Every cell is from a cell"*. In other words, the third postulate of cell theory states that all cells are formed only by the division of other cells. The modern content of the cell theory can be summarised as follows: the *basic structural and functional unit of living organisms is the cell.* The cell theory is the most important achievement of natural science. It has played an outstanding role in the development of not only biology and medicine, but also many other sections of human science.
At present, the basic tenets of the cell theory are formulated as follows:
1) The cell is the structural and functional unit, as well as the unit of development of all living organisms;
2) the cell has an inherent membrane structure;
3) the nucleus is the main constituent of the cell;
4) cells only reproduce by division;
5) cellular structure - evidence that plants and animals have a common origin.
The cell theory is closely connected with the emergence and development of *cytology* (from Greek *"cytos"* - cell) - the science of cell structure, composition and functions; *cytogenetics - the* science of heredity transmission at the cellular level. A major step forward was the invention of the electron microscope by Zworykin and the phase-contrast microscope by F. Zernike in the 30s. Magnification of 100 thousand and more times, which is able to give electron microscope, allows you to see the smallest details of the structure of cell organoids. Modern achievements of cytology are associated with the use of physical (method of labelled atoms) and chemical methods. As is known, all living organisms due to their inherent primary property of heredity, retain in a number of generations characteristic for them features, that is, reproduce similar to themselves and pass this continuity from generation to generation in the process of reproduction.
The cell is the basis of the structure of any organism, and in reproduction it is the link between two generations. Cells of different 13

of organisms and in different tissues are very diverse in size, shape, structure and function, but the general scheme of cell structure is the same. The basic elements of all cells are membrane, cytoplasm and nucleus.

Cell Membrane. Each cell is covered by a *plasma (cytoplasmic) membrane* that is 8-12 nm thick. This membrane is built of two layers of lipids (bilipid layer, or bilayer). Each lipid molecule is formed by a hydrophilic head and a hydrophobic tail. In biological membranes, lipid molecules are arranged with their heads facing outwards and their tails facing inwards (towards each other).

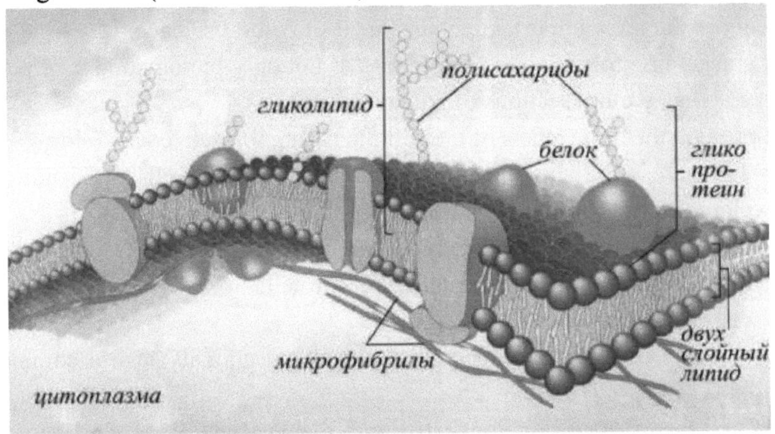

Figure 1. Structure of the cell membrane.

The double layer of lipids provides a barrier function of the membrane, preventing the cell contents from spreading and preventing dangerous substances from entering the cell. Numerous protein molecules are embedded in the bilipid layer of the membrane.

One is on the outside of the membrane, others are on the inside, and others permeate the entire membrane. Membrane proteins are called *receptors.* With their help, the cell perceives various influences on its surface. Other proteins form channels through which various ions are transported into and out of the cell. Third proteins are enzymes that ensure the processes of vital activity in the cell (Fig. 1).

Cytoplasm. The obligatory part of the cell enclosed between the plasma membrane and the nucleus. Cytoplasm of an animal cell

- A complexly organised system that represents the bulk of the cell. It consists of a colloidal solution of proteins and other organic substances: 85% of this solution is water, 10% proteins and 5% other compounds. The cytoplasm is heterogeneous in structure. Cytoplasm includes various organoids. The space between them is filled with *cytosol - a* viscous aqueous solution of various salts and organic substances, penetrated by a system of protein filaments - *cytoskeleton.* It consists of three elements: *microtubules, intermediate filaments and microfilaments.*

Microtubules permeate the entire cytoplasm and are hollow tubes with a diameter of 20-30 nm. Their walls are formed by specially twisted threads made of tubulin protein. The assembly of microtubules from tubulin takes place in the *cell centre.* Microtubules are strong and form the supporting framework of the cytoskeleton. They are often arranged to counteract cell stretching and contraction. In addition to their mechanical function, microtubules also fulfil a transport function, participating in the transport of various substances through the cytoplasm. Intermediate filaments are about 10 nm thick and are also proteinaceous. Their functions are currently insufficiently studied.

Microfilaments are protein fil**aments** with a diameter of only 4 nm. They are based on the protein actin. Sometimes actin filaments are grouped into bundles. Microfilaments are most often located close to the plasma membrane and are able to change its shape, which is very important, for example, for the processes of phagocytosis and pinocytosis.

The cytoplasm is composed of the following organoids: endoplasmic network, ribosomes, mitochondria, Golgi complex, lysosomes, peroxisomes, and others. (Figure 2). Most of the chemical and physiological processes of the cell take place in the cytoplasm. Newly synthesised proteins and other substances move within the cell or are excreted from the cell.

Endoplasmic network or reticulum. A distinction is made between *smooth endoplasmic reticulum* (ER) and *rough endoplasmic reticulum* (RER). HER is a system of smooth intracellular membranes: this organelle contains enzymes that neutralise toxic substances (oxidases in particular). Lipid synthesis and hydrolytic cleavage of glycogen occur on HER membranes. HER is a system of intracellular membranes with numerous attached 15
ribosomes, which give the appearance of roughness. A part of the SER is in direct contact with the nuclear membrane. Different types of proteins

are synthesised on the membranes of hERs.

Ribosomes are complexly organised submicroscopic granules located on the membranes of the endoplasmic network or freely in the cytoplasm. Ribosomes can be single or united in complexes - *polyribosomes.* They are composed of proteins and high molecular weight RNA in approximately equal proportions. The function of ribosomes is the synthesis of proteins of the organism. Disc-shaped membranes and numerous vesicles associated with them represent the so-called Golgi complex.

The Golgi apparatus accumulates various products of cellular metabolism and external substances. Its loops concentrate substances into droplets or granules, which are then excreted outside the cell.

Mitochondria. These are spherical rod-shaped formations of complex structure. They consist of a matrix surrounded by an inner membrane, an intermembrane space and an outer membrane.

Matrix is the main homogeneous or fine-grained substance of the cell, filling the intracellular space between the cristae - bulging inner membrane. The matrix contains circular DNA molecules, specific RNA, and granules of calcium and magnesium salts.

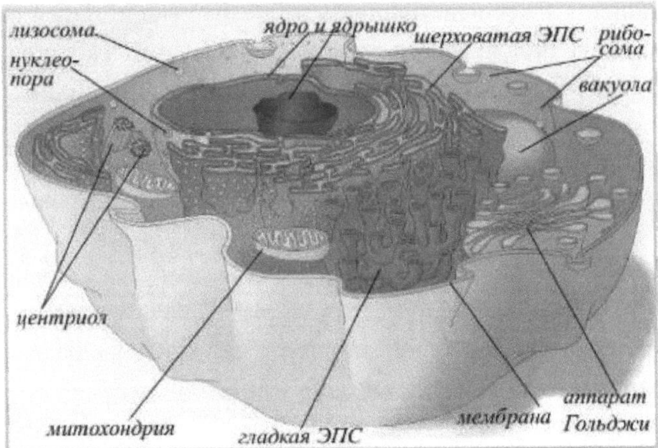

Figure 2. The structure of a cell.

Membranes are composed of proteins and phospholipids. Mitochondria are capable of self-reproduction. In mitochondria due to oxidative 16 energy is produced in the form of ATP (adenosine triphosphate) molecules. Cellular respiration takes place with the participation of mitochondria.

The cytoplasm of the cell contains *lysosomes.* They look like membrane-covered sacs and contain enzymes that break down nucleic acids, proteins, and polysaccharides. Lysosomes are the *"digestive system" of* the cell. In case of membrane disruption, lysosomes can also digest the contents of the cell cytoplasm - autolysis (self-digestion).

The peroxisomes of the cell are oval-shaped corpuscles bounded by a membrane and located on both sides of the reticulum.

Peroxisomes contain a granular matrix with crystal-like structures consisting of fibrils and tubes in the centre. The contents of peroxisomes are amino acid oxidation enzymes and catalase. The metabolism of amino acids produces hydrogen peroxide H2O2, which is broken down by catalase. Thus, peroxisome catalase has a protective function as $H_2 O_2$ is a toxic compound to the cell.

The centrosome, or **"cell centre", is** usually located in the centre of the cell or near the nucleus. It consists of two *centrioles* located in a specially organised area of the cytoplasm. The centrosome participates in the process of cell division by creating the division spindle. Sometimes inclusions are identified in the cytoplasm of the cell. They are not an obligatory component, as they represent various metabolic products (crystals of uric acid salts, pigment grains, fats, proteins, etc.) and can be utilised by the organism if necessary.

Cell nucleus. The nucleus is the most important structure in eukaryotic cells. It represents the control centre of the cell and the storage of information about it. More than 90% of cellular DNA, a substance that carries hereditary information, is localised in the nucleus. Usually the nucleus is one, but there can be binuclear and even multinuclear cells (for example, some human liver cells, transverse striated muscle fibres). The shape of the nucleus is more often round or oval and is usually determined by the shape of the cell and its function. In some cell types, nuclei are flattened (e.g., endothelial cells) or segmented (e.g., human neutrophil leukocytes). The size of the nucleus in different cell types varies and is highly dependent on the functional activity of the cell.

The structure of the nucleus varies in different periods of cell life. In interphase cells (the period when cells do not divide), all nuclei are characterised by the presence of a shell, chromatin, nucleus and nuclear juice - *karyoplasm.*

The ***nuclear envelope*** is formed by two membranes (inner and outer), between which there is a gap - the perinuclear space. The perinuclear space communicates with EPS channels, and the outer membrane of the nuclear envelope is similar in structure to the membranes of granular EPS. The nuclear envelope contains pores through which various macromolecules selectively pass. The nuclear envelope separates the internal environment of the nucleus from the cytoplasm and regulates the flow of substances from the cytoplasm into the nucleus and vice versa.

The ***nucleus*** is usually intensely coloured and has a compact structure. The nucleus may contain a single nucleus or several nuclei. The electron microscope reveals the connection of the nucleus with chromosome sections - nucleus organisers. These sites are used for the synthesis of ribosomal RNA (rRNA). In the nucleus, rRNA forms a complex with protein and ribosomes are formed.

The ***chromatin of*** the nucleus is in the form of granules or clumps that are intensively stained with special dyes. This staining is due to the presence of DNA and proteins in chromatin. Studies under the electron microscope revealed that chromatin is a long thin threads - ***chromosomes***, which in the dividing cell spiralise and become dense and short corpuscles. Thanks to this, the chromosomes of dividing cells are clearly distinguishable in the light microscope. In other words, we can say that chromatin is interphase chromosomes in a despiralised state. In the interphase nucleus, not all the chromatin is visible, but only those parts of it that remain spiralised in the non-dividing cell.

1.2. STRUCTURE AND FUNCTIONS OF CHROMOSOMES. HUMAN KARYOTYPE

The concepts of chromosomes were first introduced by the German morphologist W.Waldeyer (1888) and proposed to call them *chromosomes* (from Greek *chromatos* - colour + *soma* - body) because they were intensely coloured by some dyes . *Chromosomes* can be located in spiralised and despiralised form. During interphase, the chromosomes are almost invisible because they are despiralised.

Only after staining with special dyes do they become visible. Chromosomes that are in the interphase period are called *chromatin.*

When metaphase plates are analysed under a light microscope, it can be distinguished that any chromosome consists of two *arms and a centromere*, or *primary tether*, which acts as the mechanical centre of the chromosome during division (Figure 3). The centromere is the region of the chromosome to which the filament *of the division spindle* attaches during cell *division*, propagating the chromosomes to the poles of the cell. In addition to the primary tethering, some chromosomes have a *secondary tethering* that is unrelated to the process of spindle filament attachment. The location of the secondary tether in the chromosome is associated with the formation of the nucleus, and this section of the chromosome is called the nucleus *organiser*. The genes responsible for rRNA synthesis are located in the nucleus organisers. The function of the other secondary tethers is not yet clear. The section of chromatid between the centromere and telomere is called the arm.

The long arm of a chromosome is denoted by the Latin letter "q", the short arm by **"p".** If the centromere is located in the centre of the chromosome and as if divides it into equal parts, such a chromosome is called equal-shouldered or *metacentric* (1st and 16th chromosomes) (Fig. 4). If one shoulder is slightly larger than the other - *submetacentric* (2nd and 7th chromosomes). A chromosome with an almost terminal (terminal) centromere position, when one arm is significantly larger than the other, is called *acropentric* (13th and 21st chromosomes).

-metacentric (p = q);

-submetacentric (q> p);

-acrocentric (one-shouldered - q).

Some acrocentric chromosomes have so-called satellites - regions connected to the rest of the chromosome by a thin strand of chromatin.

Such chromosomes are called *satellite* chromosomes. The size of the satellite relative to the length of the whole chromosome is constant for each particular chromosome. In the human karyotype, five pairs of chromosomes have satellites: 13th, 14th, 15th, 21st and 22nd.

The ends of chromosomes have segments that prevent the chromosomes from sticking together at their ends and thus help to maintain their integrity. These segments have been called *telomeres*.

Therefore, telomeres are responsible for the existence of chromosomes as individual entities. Chromosomes that have the same order of genes are called *homologous*. They have the same structure (length, centromere location, etc.). *Non-homologous* chromosomes have different gene sets and different structures.

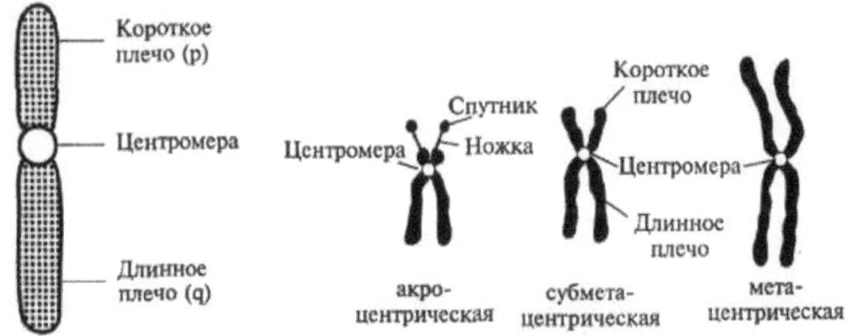

Fig.Z. Schematic representation of a chromosome.

Figure 4. Dependence of chromosome shape on centromere position.

The study of the fine structure of chromosomes has shown that they are composed of DNA, protein (mainly histones) and a small amount of RNA. The different parts of chromosomes are heterogeneous. Those parts that stain more intensely are called *heterochromatin.* They have the appearance of a helix and are in an almost inactive state. The poorly stained parts of chromosomes are called *euchromatin.* They are despiralised sections of chromosomes and consist of genes in the active state. The size of the DNA molecule of chromosomes is enormous. Each chromosome is represented by a single DNA molecule. They can reach hundreds of micrometres and even centimetres. Of the human chromosomes, the largest is the first chromosome; its DNA has a total length of up to 7 cm. The total length of the DNA molecule of all the chromosomes of a single human cell is 170 cm. Despite their gigantic size, DNA molecules function within micro formations such as chromosomes. Therefore, the chromosomes of cell nuclei must be highly shortened (condensed) DNA structures.

This is achieved due to the specific stacking of DNA molecules - multilevel helicalisation. This specific stacking of chromosomal DNA is provided by histone proteins. Histones are arranged along the length of the DNA molecule in the form of blocks. One block contains 8 histone molecules, forming a *nucleosome* (a formation consisting of a DNA strand wound around a histone octamer). The main structural unit of the chromosome is the nucleosome, The size of the nucleosome is about 10 nm. Nucleosomes look like beads strung on a string.

Nucleosomes and the DNA sections connecting them are tightly packed in the form of a helix, with six nucleosomes per turn of such a helix. This is how the structure of a chromosome is formed (Fig. 5).

Each nucleosome contains two molecules of four different types of histones combined into an octamer (octahedron) wrapped in a DNA strand. Nucleosomes and the DNA sections connecting them form a helical structure - a chromatin fibre. There are 6 nucleosomes for each turn of such a helix. This is how the structure of the chromosome is formed (Fig. 6). Such organisation allows to pack a very long DNA molecule into a compact structure. Condensation reduces the length of the DNA molecule by a factor of 10,000, so that condensed chromosomes are on average about 200 nm long (i.e. 200x10-9 m). This provides the possibility of precise and rapid division of the genetic material of the mother cell between daughter cells (mitosis) and halving the number of chromosomes during the formation of germ cells (meiosis).

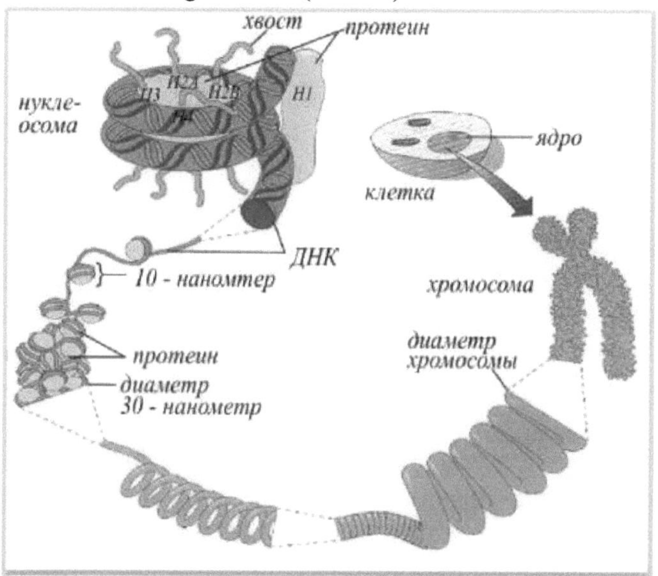

Figure 5. Structure of nucleosomes and their relationship to the chromosome and DNA molecule (in the metaphase chromosome).

Chromosomes function as the basic genetic apparatus of the cell. They contain ***genes*** in a linear order, each of which occupies a strictly defined location called a locus.

Alternative forms of a gene (i.e. its different states) occupying the same locus are called alleles (from Greek *allelon* - mutually different, other). Any chromosome contains only a single allele at a given locus, even though two, three or more alleles of the same gene may exist in a population.

Each species of plants and animals is characterised by its own number and morphological features of the chromosome set, i.e. a specific karyotype. The set of chromosomes of a somatic cell of a particular species, characterised by the number, size and shape of chromosomes, is called *karyotype.*

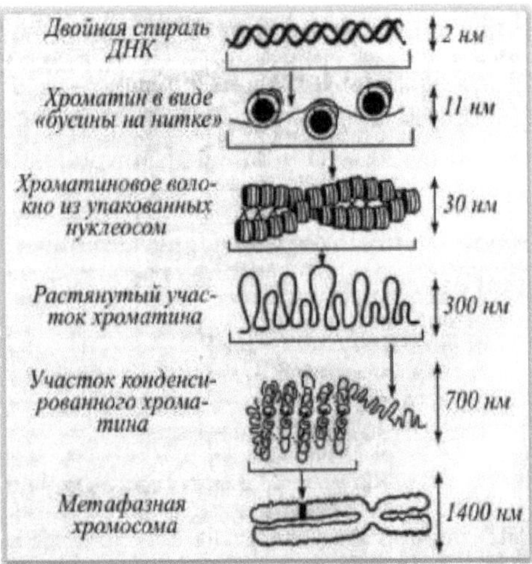

Figure 6. General scheme of chromosome structure.

The number of chromosomes in mature germ cells is called *haploid* and is denoted by the Latin letter "*p*". Somatic cells contain a double number of chromosomes, which is called the *diploid set,* denoted by "*2p*". Cells that have more than two sets of chromosomes are called *polyploid (4p, 8p, 16p, etc.).* Paired chromosomes, i.e., identical in shape, structure, and size but of different origins (one is maternal, the other paternal), are called homologous. The number of chromosomes in the karyotype is not related to the level of organisation of living organisms: primitive forms may have a greater number of chromosomes than highly organised ones, and vice versa. For example, radiolaria cells contain 1000 - 1600 chromosomes, while chimpanzee cells contain only 48. However, it should be remembered that all organisms of the same species have the same number of chromosomes, i.e. they are characterised by species specificity of the karyotype.

The imperfection of the applied methods of analysis made the study of chromosomes difficult. It is this circumstance that for a long time prevented the determination of the true number of chromosomes in human cells.

Only in 1956 two cytogeneticists - American J.Tiyo and Swede A.Levan, having improved the technique of preparation of chromosome preparations, proved that normal somatic cells of a human being contain 46 chromosomes forming 23 homologous pairs; 22 pairs of chromosomes identical in men and women were called autosomal chromosomes (autosomes); the 23rd pair of chromosomes differing in men and women was called a pair of sex chromosomes.

In females, sex chromosomes are represented by two identical (homologous) chromosomes (XX), in males by chromosomes that differ in size and shape (X and Y).

The **karyotype** is the passport of a species. Karyotype analysis allows the detection of abnormalities that can lead to developmental anomalies, hereditary diseases or death of foetuses and embryos in the early stages of development.

1.3. CLASSIFICATION AND FINE STRUCTURE OF CHROMOSOMES

Human chromosomes differ in size, centromere location, and secondary strands. The karyotype was first subdivided into groups in 1960 at a conference in Denver (USA). The description of the human karyotype was initially based on the following two principles: chromosome arrangement by length; chromosome grouping by centromere location (metacentric, submetacentric, acrocentric).

According to the classification, all human chromosomes are divided into 7 groups, arranged in decreasing order of their length, and are designated by letters of the English alphabet from A to G.

All pairs of chromosomes began to be numbered with Arabic numerals.

Group A (1-3rd) are the largest chromosomes. The 1st and 3rd are metacentric, the 2nd is submetacentric.

Group B (4th and 5th) are large submetacentric chromosomes.

Group C (6th-12th and X chromosome) are medium-sized submetacentric chromosomes.

Group D (13th-15th)-acrocentric chromosomes of medium size.

Group E (16th -18th) are small submetacentric chromosomes.

Group P (19th and 20th) are the smallest metacentric chromosomes.

The *Q group* (21st, 22nd and Y) are the smallest acrocentric chromosomes.

The proposed classification allowed a clear distinction between chromosomes belonging to different groups (Figure 7).

Figure 7. Human karyotype. (XX females and XU males

have 46 chromosomes each).

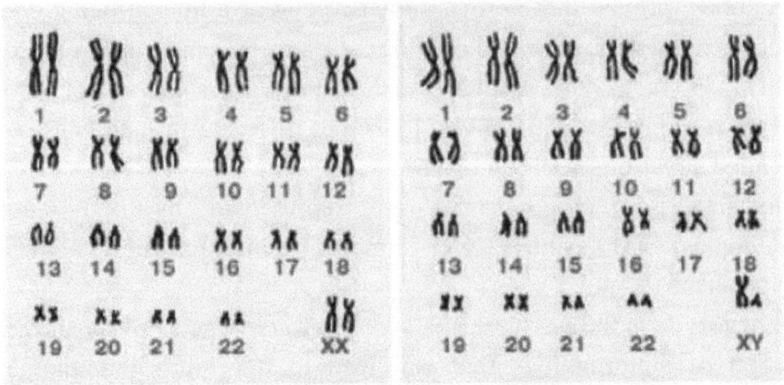

In subsequent years, the chromosome classification was supplemented with data on the position of secondary tethers. However, the needs of clinical practice showed that the proposed group Denver and refined London classifications of chromosomes are insufficient for individual identification of chromosomes.

Knowledge of the molecular structure of chromosomes became the basis for the development of methods of differential staining of chromosomes, which is based on the use of dyes that specifically bind to DNA sites of a certain structure, this allowed to identify each chromosome. Moreover, the identification of chromosomes is carried out not by individual random features, but actually, by their structural and functional organisation. Different researchers have proposed different methods for identifying linear heterogeneity (segmentation) of individual chromosomes.

In 1971, at the Paris Conference on Standardisation and Nomenclature of Human Chromosomes, all these methods were compared and it was shown that they detected essentially the same chromosome regions or segments. The different segments were labelled according to the methods and dyes with which they were best detected:

Q - Segments (quinacrine, acrychin);

G - Segments (Giemza, Giemza);

R - Segments (reverse, negotiable);

C - Segments (constitutive heterochromatin).

It should be emphasised that with all the variety of chromosome treatments with different dyes used, the linear heterogeneity of chromosomes detected is always the same. The use of methods of differential staining of chromosomes made it possible to "recognise" each chromosome and widely use this technique in clinical cytogenetics (Fig. 8).

It can be clearly seen that each human chromosome has a sequence of differently broad bands unique to it. This makes it possible to accurately identify any of the chromosomes and detect relatively large changes in their structure. When analysing *metaphase chromosomes* of average condensation, about 350 to 400 relatively large segments per haploid set can be clearly distinguished. In the stages preceding metaphase, chromosomes are less spiralled and therefore have greater transverse subdivision. Methods have been developed to analyse chromosomes on dividing cells at the *prometaphase* stage. Using this methodological approach, chromosomes with varying degrees of segmentation, ranging from 800 to 2500 segments per haploid set, were obtained. Differentially stained X and Y chromosomes with different levels of helicalisation are shown in (Figure 9). The approach used makes it possible to accurately identify breakpoints in rearranged chromosomes, even if small chromosome segments are involved in rearrangement.

Transverse striation, detected by different methods, in principle reveals the same segments of the chromosome and is the result of uneven condensation of chromatin along its entire length. Depending on the degree of DNA spiralisation in the chromosome, *heterochromatin and euchromatin* regions are distinguished, which are characterised by different functional and genetic properties.

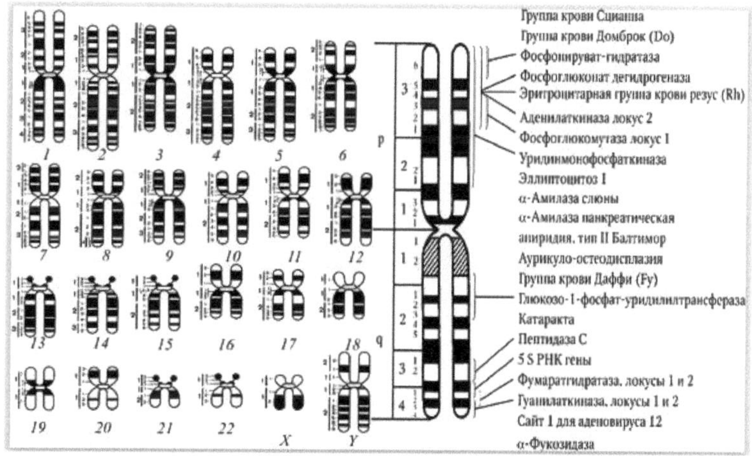

Figure 8. Human chromosomes in G staining.

Figure 9. Differentially stained ChiU chromosomes with different levels of helicalisation.

The heterochromatin region is an area of condensed chromatin (highly heterochromatinised DNA), which can be detected by differential staining as dark bands. The presence of heterochromatin can also be detected in the interphase nucleus, where it is clearly identified as intensely stained clumps of chromatin. Reading of genetic information from these sites does not occur. A distinction *is made between structural and facultative* heterochromatin. Structural heterochromatin is constantly present in certain regions of the chromosome. For example, it is always found around the centromeres of all chromosomes. Facultative heterochromatin appears in the chromosome when euchromatin regions become supercoiled. Facultative heterochromatisation may involve an entire chromosome. Thus, in the cells of the female organism, one of the X chromosomes is completely inactivated by heterochromatisation already at the early stages of embryonic development. It can be detected as a clump of heterochromatin on the periphery of the nucleus. Such an inactivated X chromosome is called sex chromatin or Barr's corpuscles (Fig. 10).

Due to heterochromatisation of the X chromosome in female cells, the number of genes functioning in male and female cells is equalised, as males have only one X chromosome.

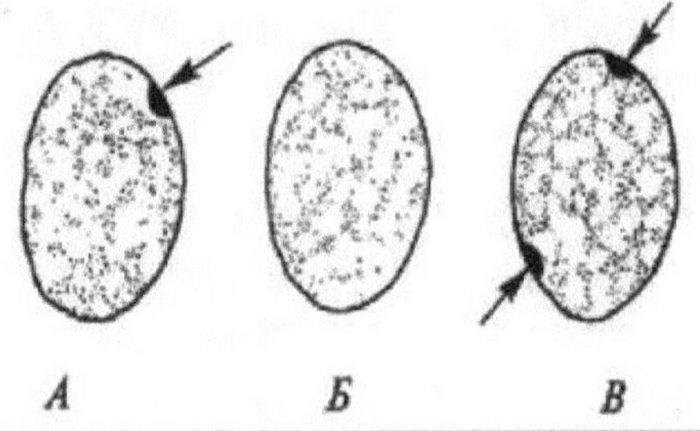

Fig. 10. Cells of the oral mucosa: A- there is one Barr's corpuscle in a female cell; B- there are no Barr's corpuscles in a male cell; C- there are two Barr's corpuscles in a male cell with chromosomal abnormality (XXXU).

The euchromatin regions of chromosomes in the interphase nucleus are not visible because they are represented by chromatin in a decondensed state. This indicates their high metabolic activity. Indeed, euchromatin regions contain unique genes controlling the synthesis of various proteins. In differential staining of metaphase chromosomes, they are defined as light bands.

1.4. REPRODUCTION OF ORGANISMS

Every second on Earth, an astronomical number of living beings die of old age, disease and predators, and it is only through reproduction, this universal property of organisms, that life on Earth does not cease.

Reproduction is one of the most important properties of living organisms. It may seem that the processes of reproduction in living things are very diverse, but all of them can be reduced to two forms: sexless and sexual. Methods of reproduction in different organisms can vary greatly, but the basis of any type of reproduction is cell division. New cells arise from the division of existing cells. When a unicellular organism divides, two new organisms arise from the old (mother) organism. A multicellular organism develops from a single cell: its numerous offspring arise by repeated cell divisions. This process continues throughout life: as cells grow and develop, and as they regenerate, repairing (replacing) the cells that have served their purpose.

The discovery of the fundamental law, formulated by R. Virchow (1855), that every cell is derived from a cell, initiated a close study of the processes of cell division. In 1882, W. Fleming reported that during cell nucleus division, chromosomes (the term itself was proposed later) divide lengthwise. A year later, E. Van Beneden drew attention to the fact that the chromosomes distributed among daughter cells exactly repeat the structure of the maternal old chromosome. At the same time, E. Strasburger, W. Roux and O. Getwig formulated *the "nuclear hypothesis of heredity".*

Thus, material continuity in the series of cellular generations of individuals is accomplished by the reproduction of organisms, the central point of which is cell division.

1.5. CELL DIVISION - MECHANISM OF HEREDITARY PROPERTIES CONTINUITY

The ability to divide is the most important property of cells. Without division it is impossible to imagine an increase in the number of unicellular creatures, the development of a complex multicellular organism from a single fertilised egg, the renewal of cells, tissues and even organs lost in the process of vital activity of the organism.

Cell division is carried out in stages. At each stage of division, certain processes take place. They lead to the doubling of genetic material (DNA synthesis) and its distribution among daughter cells. The period of a cell's life from one division to the next is called the *cell cycle,* which thus consists of a stage of relative rest, or *interphase*, and cell division. During interphase, the chromosomes are in a despiralised (unwound) state and are therefore not visible under a light microscope. This is why, at first, researchers assumed that the nucleus, which is in a non-dividing state, is at rest. In fact, it is during interphase that the nucleus is most active in metabolic (metabolic and synthetic) processes, and the cell performs its usual functions or prepares for subsequent division.

Preparation for division. Eukaryotic organisms, consisting of cells with nuclei, begin preparation for division at a certain stage of the cell cycle, in *interphase.* It is during interphase that the process of protein biosynthesis takes place in the cell, and all the most important structures of the cell are doubled.

If the number of chromosomes in the haploid (single) set is denoted as "p" and the amount of DNA as **"c"**, then the diploid (double) set of genetic material will have "2p2c", respectively. The preparation of a cell for division consists of three periods. Immediately after the preceding division, the cell enters the G1-beginning of interphase period.

The presynthetic period (G1) is the longest part of interphase. It can last from 2-3 hours to several days in different cell types. This period follows immediately after the preceding division, during which the cell grows, accumulating energy and substances for the subsequent DNA doubling.

The synthetic period (S) - which is usually divided 6-10 hours, includes DNA doubling - this is the replication (doubling) of the amount of DNA (2p4s), proteins needed to form chromosomes, and an increase in the amount of RNA. By the end of this period, each chromosome already consists of two identical chromatids joined together at the centromere region. During the same period, centrioles double in size.

The post-synthetic period (G2) occurs after chromosome doubling. It lasts 2-5 h. During this time, energy is accumulated for the upcoming mitosis and microtubule proteins are synthesised, which subsequently form the division spindle (2p4c). The cell can now proceed to mitosis. Actually, mitotic division occupies only a minor part of the cell cycle. Interphase in plant and animal cells on average lasts 10-20 hours. Then comes the process of cell division - *mitosis.*

Phases of mitosis. Mitosis, or indirect division, is the division of the nucleus that results in the formation of two daughter nuclei, each of which has exactly the same set of chromosomes as the parent nucleus. The division of the nucleus is usually followed by the division of the cell itself, so the term "mitosis" often refers to the division of the entire cell.

Mitosis was first observed in plaunal spores by I.D. Chistyakov in 1874. Detailed studies of the behaviour of chromosomes in mitosis were carried out by the German botanist E. Strasburger in 1879 on plants and by the German histologist W. Flemming in 1882 on animals, who observed the appearance and described the behaviour of filamentous structures in the nucleus during division. Hence the name of the division process - mitosis (from Greek *mitos* - thread). During mitotic division, the cell nucleus undergoes a series of strictly ordered sequential changes with the formation of specific filamentous structures. Mitosis includes two processes: division of the nucleus *(karyokinesis)* and division of the cytoplasm *(cytokinesis)*. Mitosis is divided into four consecutive phases: prophase, metaphase, anaphase and telophase.

Prophase is the first stage of preparation for division. DNA spiralisation occurs in the nucleus; tightly twisted chromosomes are clearly visible in the microscope. During this period, the double nature of the chromosomes can be observed, as each chromosome appears longitudinally doubled. These chromosome halves (the result of chromosome reduplication (doubling) in 3-phase), called sister chromatins, are held together by one common region, the centromere. The centrioles begin to diverge towards the poles and the microtubules branching from them begin to form the *division spindle* (2p4c). Nuclei disappear. The nuclear envelope is destroyed and the mixing of karyoplasm with cytoplasm begins. Mixoplasm is formed, which facilitates the movement of chromosomes to the equatorial plane of the cell (Fig. 11).

Metaphase. Chromosomes are arranged in such a way that their centromeres are in the plane of the cell equator. The so-called metaphase plate, consisting of chromosomes, is formed. At the metaphase stage, the chromosomes have the shortest length because at this time they are most strongly spiralled and condensed. This stage is most suitable for counting the number of chromosomes in a cell, studying and describing their structure, determining their size, etc. The arrangement of the chromosomes in relation to each other is random. The division spindle is fully formed and the strands of the spindle are attached to the centromeres of the chromosomes (2p4c).

Anaphase. Each chromosome longitudinally splits into two identical chromatids, which diverge to the opposite poles of the cell. Thus, due to the identity of the daughter chromatids at the two poles of the cell is the same genetic material: the same that was in the cell before the beginning of mitosis. This ensures a coordinated and accurate distribution of chromosomal material into the daughter cells (4p4c).

Telophase. The daughter chromosomes despiralise at the poles of the cell and become available for transcription. Protein synthesis begins. Nuclear envelopes and nuclei are formed.

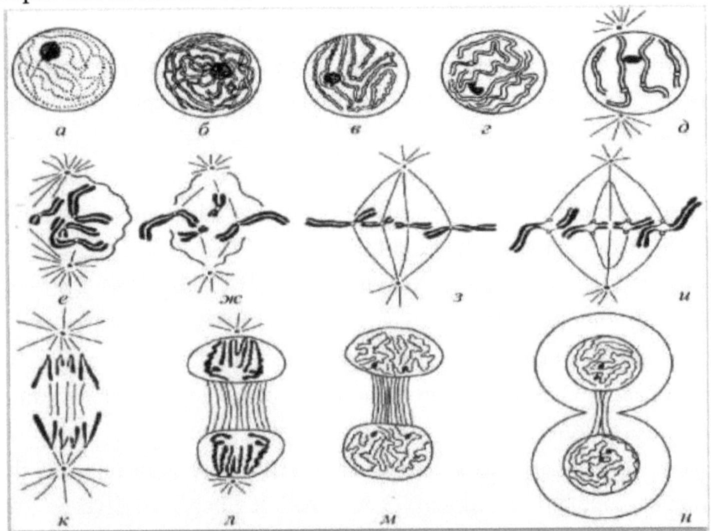

Fig. 11. Scheme of mitotic cell division: a - interphase; b, c, d, e, f, g - different stages of prophase; h, i - metaphase; j - anaphase; l, m - telophase; i - formation of two daughter cells.

The filaments of the division spindle disintegrate. This is the end of karyokinesis, and cytokinesis begins. In animal and human cells, a constriction appears in the equatorial plane. It deepens until two daughter cells separate (2p2c). Cytoskeletal structures play an important role in the formation of the constriction. From the moment of separation of daughter cells, each of them enters the interphase of a new cell cycle.

The biological significance of mitosis is as follows.

1. The events that occur during mitosis result in the formation of two genetically identical daughter cells, each containing exact copies of the genetic material of the ancestral (mother) cell.
2. Mitosis ensures the growth and development of the organism during the embryonic and post-embryonic period. The adult human body consists of approximately 1014 cells, which requires approximately 47 cycles of cell division of a single sperm fertilised egg (zygote).

3. Mitosis is a universal, evolutionarily fixed mechanism of regeneration, i.e. restoration of lost or functionally obsolete cells of the organism. It is also the basis for the processes of damage healing and sexless reproduction.

Disruption of mitosis. The proper course of mitosis can be disturbed by various external influences: high doses of radiation, some chemical substances (alcohols, esters). For example, under the influence of X-rays, the DNA of chromosomes can break. Chromosomes in this case also break. In this case, chromosomes without centromeric region may appear. Such chromosomes are unable to move in prometaphase and anaphase. In such cases, the cells will have a chromosome set that differs from the original cell. Sometimes not two but three or four poles are formed in a dividing cell, leading to three or four daughter cells respectively. In such a division, the whole well-coordinated mechanism of chromosome movement is disturbed. As a result, each daughter cell receives not the whole set of chromosomes, but only a part of it. Cells that have received an incomplete set of chromosomes, as a rule, are not viable and die.

Amitosis. In all eukaryotic organisms, the so-called *direct nuclear division* or *amitosis* is found. In amitosis there is no condensation of chromosomes or formation of a division spindle, and the nucleus divides by constriction or fragmentation, remaining in an interphase state. Cytokinesis does not always follow nucleus division, so amitosis usually results in multinucleated cells. Amitotic divisions are characteristic of cells completing the development of dying epithelial cells, ovarian follicular cells, etc. Amitosis occurs in pathological processes - inflammation, malignant growth, etc.

1.6. MEIOSIS - DIVISION, MATURATION OF SEX CELLS

The formation of sex cells (gametes) is different from the process of somatic cell reproduction. If gametes were formed in the same way, the number of chromosomes would double each time after fertilisation. However, this does not happen. Each species has a specific number of chromosomes. In sexual reproduction in plants and animals (including humans), the continuity between generations is ensured only through the sex cells - the ovum and the sperm. If the egg and sperm had the full set of genetic characteristics (2p2c) peculiar to the cells of the body, their fusion would produce an organism with a doubled set (4p4c). For example, the somatic cells of the human body contain 46 chromosomes. If a human egg and sperm each contained 46 chromosomes, when they fuse, a zygote with

92 chromosomes would be formed.

The next generation would show descendants with 184 chromosomes, etc. At the same time, it is well known that the number of chromosomes is a strict species characteristic, and a change in their number leads either to the death of the organism at the early stages of embryonic development or causes severe diseases. Thus, during the formation of germ cells, there must be a mechanism that leads to a reduction in the number of chromosomes by exactly half. This process is *meiosis* (from Greek *meiosis* - reduction).

Sexual reproduction emerged in the process of evolution as the highest form of reproduction of organisms, allowing to repeatedly increase the number of offspring, and, most importantly, sexual reproduction was a necessary prerequisite for the emergence of many forms of hereditary variability. These two factors largely contributed to the natural selection of the most adapted individuals and thus significantly determined the speed of evolutionary transformations.

A special type of cell division resulting in the formation of sex cells is called *meiosis*. In each division of meiosis, by analogy with mitosis, a prophase, metaphase, anaphase and telophase are distinguished. Unlike mitosis, in which the number of chromosomes produced by the daughter cells is maintained, meiosis halves the number of chromosomes in the daughter cells.

The process of meiosis consists of two consecutive cell divisions - meiosis I and meiosis II. DNA and chromosome doubling occurs only before meiosis I. The first division of meiosis, called the *reduction* division, results in cells with the number of chromosomes halved. The second division of meiosis, called the *equational division, is* followed by the formation of mature germ cells. In each division of meiosis, by analogy with mitosis, a prophase, metaphase, anaphase and telophase are distinguished.

The most complex stage of meiosis is prophase I. It consists of the following stages: leptonema, zygonema, pachynema, diplonema and diakinesis. DNA synthesis, which started in interphase, continues in prophase I, which is not found in mitosis (Fig. 12).

The earliest stage of prophase I, *leptonema* (or called *leptotene* in some textbooks), does not differ from the prophase of mitosis. In this stage, thin twisted strands of chromosomes appear. Chromosome filaments during this period are mostly single, but sometimes bifurcated at the ends (sister chromatids).

At the *zygoneme* stage, *conjugation* (each chromosome "finds" a homologous chromosome and converges with it) occurs, first of all, in separate parts of homologous chromosomes, and then along the entire length. The conjugated pair of chromosomes is called a *bivalent.* It has four chromatids, but they are not yet distinguishable microscopically.

The pachynema stage is characterised by a haploid number of bivalents. The chromatids of each chromosome, the sister chromosomes, are already clearly visible.

At the pachynema stage, one can see nuclei attached to certain parts of chromosomes in the region of secondary strands. In *diplonema,* the structures of bivalents and the four chromatids composing them are clearly revealed. The bivalent is therefore called a tetrad at this time. Reduplicated homologues are repelled from each other.

Non-sister chromatids can be connected to each other at some points, forming a figure in the form of a Greek letter (%). Therefore, the crossing points are called *chiasms.* Chiasms indicate the exchange of sections of homologous chromosomes in a bivalent. This phenomenon is called *crossingover.*

Further, the chromosomes forming bivalents begin to contract by spiralisation - the *diakinesis* (movement) stage. In diakinesis, the spiralisation of chromosomes increases, and the number of chiasms decreases due to movement to the ends of chromosomes. Bivalents move to the equatorial plane. The nucleus shell and nuclei disappear. The final formation of the division spindle is completed in prophase I.

A characteristic *feature of metaphase I is the* arrangement of homologous chromosomes in pairs in the equatorial plane of the cell. This is followed by *anaphase I,* during which whole homologous chromosomes, each consisting of two chromatids, diverge to the opposite poles of the cell. It is very important to emphasise one feature of chromosome divergence at this stage of meiosis: the homologous chromosomes of each pair diverge randomly, independently of the chromosomes of other pairs. At each pole there are half as many chromosomes as there were in the cell at the beginning of division. Then comes *telophase I,* during which two cells with halved number of chromosomes are formed.

The very short period of time between the first and second meiosis is called ***interkinesis.*** In interkinesis, no doubling of the number of DNA molecules is required. The second meiotic division (meiosis II) follows. It differs from mitosis only in that the number of chromosomes in ***metaphase II*** is half the number of chromosomes in the metaphase of mitosis in the same organism. Since each chromosome consists of two chromatids, in metaphase II the chromosome centromeres divide and chromatids diverge to the poles, which become daughter chromosomes. Only now comes the real interphase. Four cells with a haploid set of chromosomes arise from each initial cell.

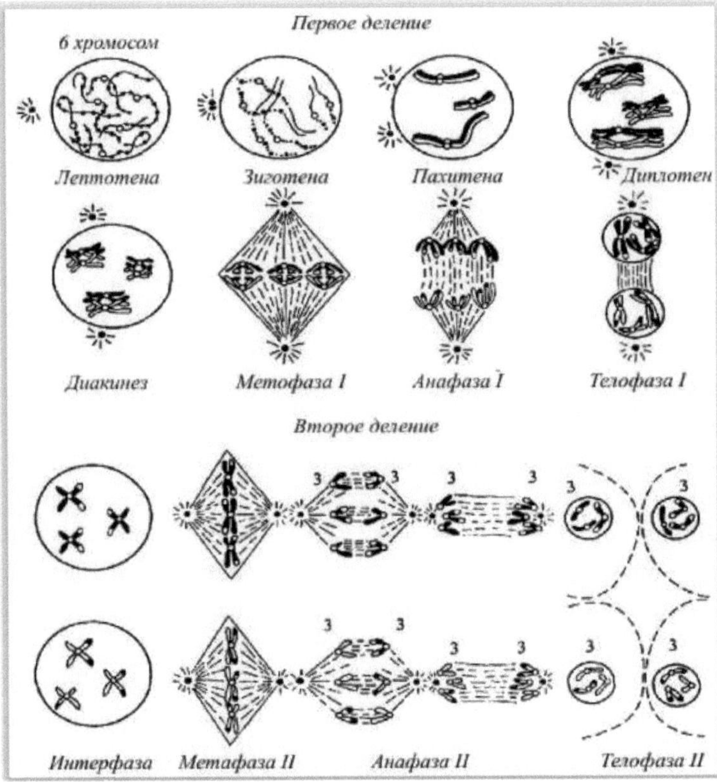

Figure 12: The first and second divisions of meiosis.

Thus, a diploid cell that has entered meiosis forms four daughter cells with a haploid set of chromosomes.

The biological significance of meiosis is as follows:

1. Meiosis provides continuity in a series of generations of sexually reproducing organisms, while mitosis performs the same task in a series of cellular generations.
2. Meiosis is one of the most important steps in the process of sexual reproduction.

3. During meiosis, there is a reduction in the number of chromosomes from the diploid number (46 in humans) to the haploid number (23).

4. Meiosis provides combinative hereditary variability, which is a prerequisite for the genetic diversity of humans and the genetic uniqueness of each individual. Combinatorial genetic variability during meiosis results from two events: random distribution of non-homologous chromosomes and crossingover, i.e. mutual exchange of homologous chromatid regions during the formation of chiasms.

5. Meiosis is called maturation division because the formation of human sex cells (gametes), like other eukaryotes, involves a reduction in the number of chromosomes.

1.7. GERM CELL DEVELOPMENT. FERTILISATION

Sexual reproduction involves, as a rule, two parental individuals, each of which participates in the formation of a new organism, contributing only one sex cell - ***gamete*** (egg or sperm), which has half the number of chromosomes than non-sex, i.e. somatic, cells of the parents. As a result of the fusion of gametes, a fertilised ovum - ***zygote*** - is formed, carrying the hereditary characteristics of both parents, thus dramatically increasing the hereditary variability of the offspring. This is the advantage of sexual reproduction over sexual reproduction.

The process of formation of oocytes (female *gametes*) and spermatozoa (male *gametes*) has a common name - *gametogenesis.* In males, *spermatogenesis* occurs in the male sex glands - *testes (testis);* in females, *oocytes* are formed *(ovogenesis)* in the female sex glands - ovaries *(ovarium).*

Spermatozoa and ova are usually produced by male and female individuals, respectively. Biological species in which all organisms are divided into males and females according to the sex cells they produce are called *separate-sex* species. There are species in which the same organism has both male sex glands, the testes, and female sex glands, the ovaries. Organisms that form both kinds of sex cells are called *hermaphrodites.*

Structure of sex cells. Sex cells, or gametes, are specialised for sexual reproduction, so they are always haploid. This is their main feature. The haploidy of gametes occurs during gametogenesis, i.e. during their formation, and reflects the maturity of gametes, their readiness for fertilisation. In addition, spermatozoa and oocytes differ from somatic cells by altered nuclear-plasma relations. In oocytes, compared to somatic cells, the volume of cytoplasm is many times greater than the volume of nuclei.

Egg cells are usually the largest cells in an organism. An example is the ovum of birds. Human oocytes are spherical cells about 130-140 microns in size. The oocytes develop in the two ovaries, specialised glands of the female body located in the folds of the peritoneum.

The ovaries contain approximately 106 immature eggs by the time of birth. However, before menopause (the end of the reproductive period), only 350-400 of them mature and leave the ovaries (ovulation). Each oocyte is surrounded by follicular epithelial cells, which, as the oocyte matures, multiply and release follicular fluid that accumulates in the cavity of the primary, or primordial, follicles The functions of follicular epithelial cells are mainly to ensure the flow of nutrients - proteins, fats, amino acids - to the oocyte and the production of female sex hormones. The mature follicle, called the Graaf bubble, reaches a diameter of 2cm and protrudes beneath the surface of the ovary in the form of a tubercle. At the moment of ovulation, the wall of the Graaf bubble ruptures and the fertilising ovum is released into the abdominal cavity and enters the Fallopian tube, through which it travels to the uterine cavity. Usually only one egg is released in one of the ovaries each month.

Thus, the formation of germ cells in the female body is a cyclical process that repeats approximately every

days. It is associated with changes in the functioning and structure of the entire reproductive system of the female body (Figure 13).

Spermatozoa. Spermatozoa, or spermine, are small, mobile cells that form in the winding tubules of the male gonads (testes) after puberty. They number in the millions. The walls of the tubules consist of a number of connective tissue cells and follicular cells (Sertolli cells) that form depressions. In these recesses are located male sex cells at various stages of spermatogenesis. A mature spermatozoon consists of four main parts - head, neck, middle part and tail, or flagellum. The head of the spermatozoon contains the nucleus, which is surrounded by a thin layer of cytoplasm. Above the nucleus is a special structure, the acrosome, which contains hydrolytic enzymes that help the sperm penetrate the egg.

Two centrioles are located in the neck: the centriole closer to the nucleus is involved in the formation of the division spindle, while the other centriole is involved in the formation of the axial filament of the tail. The middle part of the spermatozoon is occupied by mitochondria assembled in a spiral around the flagellum. They provide energy for the motor activity of spermatozoa. The tail (flagellum) serves as the organ of movement (Figure 14).

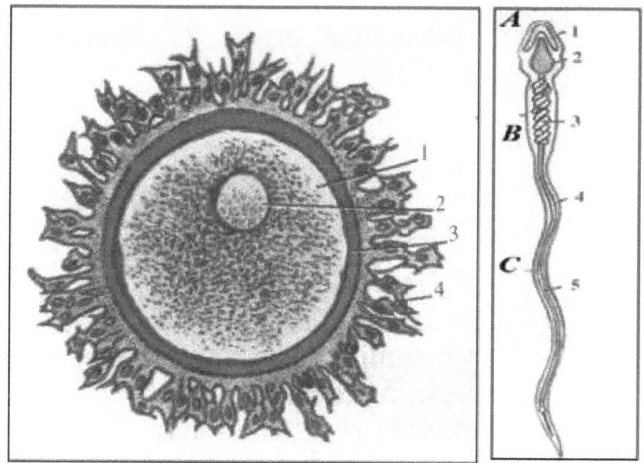

Fig. 13. Structure of the mammalian oocyte. 1 - cytoplasm; 2- nucleus; 3- primary shell;
4 - follicular cells.

Figure 14: Structure of the spermatozoon: A- head.
B-neck.
C-tail.
1- acrosome.
2- nucleus.
3-mitochondrial helix.
4- plasma membrane.
5-tail.

For example, the size of human spermatozoa is 50-70 μm. The main function of the spermatozoon is to introduce its haploid set of chromosomes into the egg during fertilisation. The structure of the spermatozoon corresponds to its functions. Most often it has a ***head*** and ***flagellum (tail),*** connected by an intermediate section - the ***neck.*** The head contains the nucleus and a special structure, the ***acrosome.***

The acrosome contains enzymes that ensure the passage of the sperm nucleus into the egg during fertilisation. In the intermediate section lie the centrioles of the cell centre and mitochondria. From the centriole comes a flagellum, which provides motility. There are also spermatozoa without flagella.

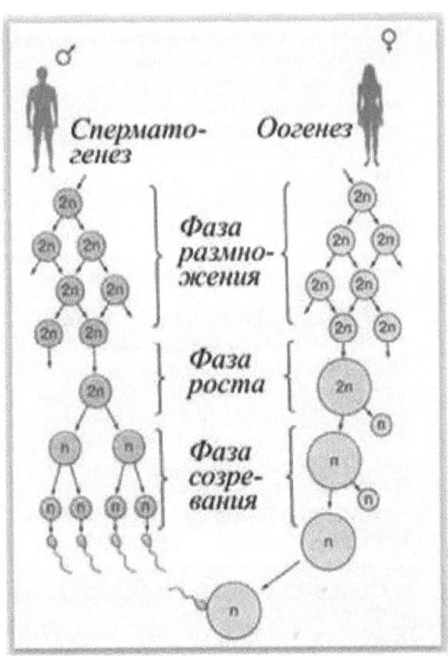

Development of sex cells (gametogenesis). Sperm cells develop in the testes, a process called *spermatogenesis.*

The process of oocyte development is called *ovogenesis* and takes place in the ovaries. Gametogenesis is divided into four stages: reproduction, growth, maturation and formation. In the *reproduction stage*, the progenitor cells with a diploid set of chromosomes reproduce by division by mitosis. This stage takes place in the germ cell reproduction zone.

In the *growth stage*, individual cells with a diploid set move to the growth zone of the sex glands and, increasing in size, accumulate nutrients, they double the amount of DNA. Then the cells, multiplying in the *maturation zone* by meiosis, form cells with haploid sets of chromosomes. In the *formation stage*, mature spermatozoa are formed.

Figure 15. Schematic of gametogenesis in humans.

This stage is absent in ovogenesis. Ovogenesis and spermatogenesis are essentially similar processes, but they have the following differences (Figure 15).

1. Ovogenesis lasts longer than spermatogenesis because the nutrients needed for the development of the foetus must be formed in the eggs.

2. In the process of spermatogenesis during meiosis, the cytoplasm is evenly distributed among all cells. During ovogenesis, it passes only to one cell and hardly passes to other cells. As a result, at the end of spermatogenesis, four cells are formed from one ancestral cell, and during ovogenesis, only one large cell is formed. The remaining three small cells

die.

3. There is no formative stage in ovogenesis.

Thus, during gametogenesis in germ cells, germ cells with a diploid (2p) set of chromosomes are formed from progenitor cells with a haploid (p) set.

Fertilisation is the process of gamete fusion. As a result of fertilisation, the chromosomes of the egg and sperm are in the same nucleus, and a *zygote, the* first cell of a new organism, *is* formed (Figure 16).

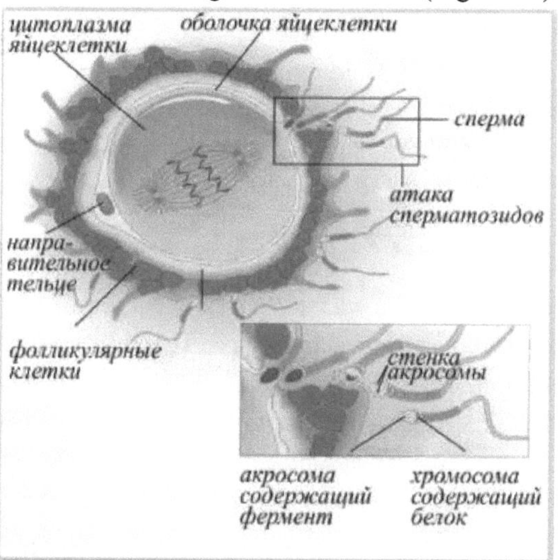

Figure 16: Fertilisation.

Spermatozoa make independent movements at a speed of 2-3 mm per minute. After 30-60 minutes, they reach the uterine cavity, and after 90-120 minutes, due to intense contractions of the uterine muscles, they get into the fallopian tubes, where they meet with eggs. Sperm retain fertilising capacity in the female genital tract for 24-48 hours. For about the same amount of time, the egg retains its fertilising capacity after ovulation. An egg is normally fertilised by only one sperm, but for fertilisation to occur, a man's seminal fluid must contain millions of sperm. The excess sperm is needed to overcome the barriers surrounding the egg.

As the sperm approaches the egg, its membrane covering the acrosome ruptures and its enzymes, hyaluronidase and protease, digest the surrounding follicular cells and the sperm penetrates the egg. Once the first (and only) sperm penetrates the egg, its membrane undergoes significant structural and functional changes that prevent other sperm from penetrating. After this, no sperm can penetrate the egg.

The sperm nucleus, moving towards the nucleus of the egg, is transformed into a male pronucleus: the chromatin, previously dense, loosens and the nuclear envelope dissolves. The penetration of the sperm into the oocyte stimulates the completion of the second division of meiosis, and the second-order ovocyte becomes a mature egg. Gradually, the male and female pronuclei converge, their membranes dissolve, and the paternal and maternal chromosomes attach to the filaments of the resulting division spindle. At this stage, the diploid number of chromosomes is restored, and the fertilised egg is called a *zygote* (from the Greek *zygotos* - connection, pair). The zygote passes through the stages of anaphase and telophase.

Subsequent division of the cytoplasm results in the formation of two diploid daughter cells. Passing through the fallopian tube into the *uterus*, the zygote undergoes a series of cell divisions, resulting in the formation of a clump of cells called a *morula* (from the Latin *morus* - mulberry) because of its resemblance to a mulberry. The resulting cells are called *blastomeres* (from Greek *blastos* - immature precursor + *meros* - part). In the morula, the inner mass of blastomeres is distinguished from the surface-lying blastomeres by cytoplasmic features and its fate. The inner group, the *embryoblast*, becomes the source of embryo development, while the outer layer forms the so-called feeding embryo. Gradually, the blastomeres are arranged around the periphery and form a wall around the central fluid-filled cavity. This stage of development is called the *blastocyst,* or *germ vesicle.* By the fourth day after fertilisation, a cluster of embryoblast cells - the germinal *node* - is formed at one of the sites of the outer layer of blastomeres, called trophoblast (from Greek *trophe* - to feed + *blastos* - immature precursor). The processes of *gastrulation* begin, during which the germinal node turns into a *germinal shield,* where the embryo body is formed.

In the uterine cavity, *trophoblast* cells multiply and by day 6-9 after fertilisation, they sink into the uterine wall, receiving nutrients from the endometrial cells (the inner, mucous layer of the uterus). This process is called implantation (from Latin *im* - in + *plantatio* - to embed). The cells of the outer layer of the trophoblast form trophoblast villi, which grow into the endometrium and provide the blastocyst with nutrients and oxygen. In later stages of development, *the placenta*, or *baby's place,* fulfils this function. The outer cells of the blastocyst form the outer membrane, or *chorion.* Two cavities appear in the inner cell mass. The cells lining these cavities form the *amnion* and the *yolk sac.* The cells comprising the inner cell mass and the yolk sac form the germinal disc from which the *embryo* subsequently develops. At an early stage, when the germinal disc is less than 2 mm in diameter, its cells differentiate into two layers - the outer layer, or *ectoderm*, and the inner layer, or *entoderm.* Later, a third germinal leaflet, *the mesoderm* (from Greek *mesos* - middle), is formed. These three germ sheets give rise to all the tissues of the developing embryo.

Most of the cells that make up the ectoderm take part in the development of the body covering and associated structures. They are used to form the external epithelium, skin glands, superficial layer of teeth, cornea, etc., which give rise to the nervous system and sensory organs. - *Ectoderm derivatives* that give rise to the nervous system and sensory organs. Cells of the inner germinal sheet, changing in conjunction with other parts of the embryo, give rise to the epithelium of the midgut, digestive glands and part of the epithelium of the respiratory system - *derivatives of the entoderm.* The *derivatives of mesoderms* are all muscular tissues, wherever they are located; all kinds of connective, cartilaginous, bone tissues, channels of excretory organs, circulatory system, part of tissues of ovaries and testes, etc. The derivatives *of mesoderms* are also *derived from mesoderms*.

The beginning of the processes of *organogenesis* (organ development) is associated with the emergence of the rudiment (laying down) of an organ, which can be caused by local changes in a certain area of a particular germinal leaflet. However, in most cases, vertebrate organs, including humans, are derived from two or all three germ sheets. In this case, the development of an organ occurs not only in the conditions of interaction between the cells composing the embryo, but also in the closest interaction between the different germ sheets.

By about the end of the 3rd week, the embryo's body systems begin to form: nervous, circulatory, digestive and other systems. In the 5th week, the rudiments of the limbs are marked. By the 8th-9th week, the laying of all organs is completed.

The first stages of development of all vertebrate embryos retain common features and are very similar, reflecting the commonality of their evolutionary history. Approximately 9-11 weeks after conception, the human embryo acquires human characteristics.

From that time until birth, it is called a *foetus.* After birth, the foetus is called a *newborn* or *infant.* The time of the organism's development from the 9th-11th week to the moment of birth is called the *antenatal period* (from Latin *ante* - before + *natalius* - birth), after which the *postnatal period* (Latin *post* - after) of life begins. The postnatal period ends with the death of the organism.

Perinatal (Greek *peri* - around) period is also distinguished, which starts from the 28th week of pregnancy, includes labour (*natal* period) and the first 7 days of the postnatal period.

Control Questions and Assignments:

1. Give a characterisation of the main organoids of the cell.
2. Give definitions of mitosis, name the phases of mitosis.
3. What is the genetic significance of mitosis?
4. Give a definition of meiosis. Name the main stages of meiosis.
5. What is the biological meaning of meiosis?
6. Describe the morphological structure of chromosomes and name their types.
7. What are the classifications of chromosomes?
8. What are the features of the structure of the ovum and sperm?
9. Into which phases is gametogenesis subdivided?
10. What is the difference between ovogenesis and spermatogenesis?

TEST-1.

1. What is a karyotype?

a) the number of nuclei in a cell;

б) the ratio of nucleus volume to nucleus volume to cytoplasm volume;

(c) Number, size and shape of chomosomes in the diploid set;

д) number, size and shape of chomosomes in a haploid set;

2. What processes occur during metaphase of fission?

a) Longitudinal division of chromosomes into chromotids and their divergence;

б) completes the movement of chromosomes to the poles;

(c) Chromosomes are in equilibrium in the region of the equator;
e) chromosomes are in equilibrium in the centromere region.

3. What is amitosis?

a) process opposite to mitosis; b) division of the nucleus without division of the cytoplasm; c) non-primate division of the nucleus and cytoplasm; e) primate division of the nucleus.

4. What is an adaptation that facilitates the process of fertilisation?

(a) yolk in the ooplasm; (b) acrosome; (c) decreased metabolism in the oocyte; (e) altered nuclear-plasmic relations;

5. What is characteristic of the crush period?

a) meiotic cell division;
б) active growth of the resulting cells;
(c) Active cellular differentiation (specialisation);
e) mitotic cell division.

CHALLENGE-1.

1. Drosophila (fruit fly) has 4 pairs of chromosomes in the nucleus of each body cell, while humans have 23 pairs. How many chromosomes will be in each daughter cell?
2. If the number of chromosomes in a diploid cell is 2p and the amount of DNA in the same cell is 2c, what will be the number of chromosomes in the amount of DNA in the cell in the anaphase I (a) and anaphase II (b) stages of meiosis.
3. As a result of fertilisation, several zygotes were formed in a Herbatceum cotton plant. Determine the number of sperm that participated in the fertilisation of the egg, if it is known that the total number of chromosomes in all the zygotes formed is 3120.
4. The total mass of all DNA molecules in 46 chromosomes of one human somatic cell is about $6\text{-}10^{-9}$ mg. Determine what will be equal to the mass of all chromosomes in one daughter cell and in two daughter cells formed by mitosis.
5. Determine the number of autosomes and sex chromosomes contained in somatic cells and in mature gametes of the following organisms:
1) Drosophila fruit fly (8); 2) mature frog (26); 3) pigeon (80); 4) chimpanzee (48); 5) human (46).
6. In the case of a human having 46 chromosomes in somatic cells, we can conventionally designate the chromosome set of female individuals by the formula 44A+XX, and of male individuals by 44A+XU (the symbol A stands for "autosomes"). Using this symbolism, write down 44

formulae for the chromosome sets of mature germ cells (gametes) formed in females and males.

7. By analogy with the previous task, make symbolic designations of chromosome sets of somatic cells and gametes of females and males of the following mammals: 1) pig (2p=40); 2) grey rat (2p=42); 3) rabbit (2p=44); 4) chimpanzee (2p=48).

CHAPTER II

HEREDITARY INFORMATION AND ITS REALISATION IN THE CELL.

2.1 INTRODUCTION

As soon as the laws of heredity were elucidated, it became obvious that genes were chemical in nature. It followed from the laws of heredity that, on the one hand, the transmission of these chemical elements from generation to generation is carried out with high precision, and on the other hand, the hereditary structures are necessarily doubled when cells multiply.

When discussing the nature of the material carriers of heredity in the 20-30s of the XX century, proteins were the first to be considered. Even the most educated geneticists considered the gene as a complex protein molecule. In 1927, the outstanding Russian biologist N.K. Koltsov formulated the principle of autocatalytic reduplication of hereditary structures.

However, the complexity of the protein molecule, which the scientist considered as a carrier of hereditary information, did not allow him to clearly develop his hypothesis to its logical conclusion.

Although DNA had been known since 1869 and its presence in chromosomes had been conclusively proven, this molecule was considered too simple to transmit hereditary information.

At the beginning of the 20th century. W.Sutton and T.Boveri suggested that chromosomes are carriers of hereditary information. Later, analysis of the chemical composition of chromosomes revealed the presence of various types of proteins and nucleic acids in their structure. Significantly greater diversity of chemical and spatial structures of proteins in comparison with nucleic acids for a long time supported the assumption about the decisive role of proteins in the transmission of hereditary information. It took several decades to be finally convinced that the material carrier of this information is only one of the constituent parts of the chromosome - *deoxyribonucleic acid (DNA)* molecule. Even experiments on mice infected with pneumococci (F. Griffith, 1928) and on microbes (O. Avery et al., 1944) only made us assume the possible participation of DNA in the transmission of hereditary properties, but were not unequivocally accepted as evidence of its determining role in the transmission of hereditary information.

It was only after the discovery of the physical and chemical structure of DNA in 1953 by J.Watson and F.Crick that it became finally clear that the transmission of hereditary information is carried out with the help of DNA.

Genetic studies of the molecular structure of chromosomes have been very fruitful. They gave an answer to two important questions: how hereditary information is stored and transmitted in cells and how hereditary information is realised. The elucidation of the structure and function of nucleic acids made it possible to understand how living organisms reproduce themselves and how genetic information is encoded, stored and realised, which is necessary for all life processes.

To date, knowledge about the structure and function of DNA has been significantly enriched, and the possibilities for research have been greatly expanded. It has been discovered that DNA can be damaged and can be repaired, that DNA molecules can exchange parts with each other, twist and untwist.

It has been shown that DNA serves as a matrix for RNA synthesis and is itself capable of being synthesised during reverse transcription with RNA. DNA functions not only in the nucleus but also in mitochondria. Currently, researchers are able to determine the sequence of nucleic bases in DNA and synthesise it.

Organisms have the ability to pass on their traits and characteristics to the next generation, i.e. to reproduce themselves. This phenomenon of trait inheritance is based on the transmission of hereditary information from generation to generation.

The material carrier of this information is the DNA molecule.

2.2. STRUCTURE AND FUNCTIONS OF NUCLEIC ACIDS

Nucleic acids. Nucleic acids were first discovered in the *nucleus*, which is the reason for their name (from Latin, *nucleus - nucleus*). They were discovered in 1869 by the Swiss chemist F. Misher in the nuclei of leukocytes.

There are two types of nucleic acids in nature, deoxyribonucleic acid (DNA) and ribonucleic acid (RNA). The difference in names is explained by the fact that the DNA molecule contains the five-carbon sugar deoxyribose, while the RNA molecule contains ribose.

At present, a large number of DNA and RNA varieties are known, differing from each other in structure and importance in metabolism. DNA is localised mainly in the chromosomes of the cell nucleus, as well as in mitochondria and chloroplasts. RNA, in addition to the nucleus, is part of ribosomes, cytoplasm, plastids and mitochondria.

Nucleic acids are complex biopolymers whose monomers are nucleotides. Each nucleotide consists of a five carbon sugar (ribose or deoxyribose), a nitrogenous base and a phosphoric acid residue.

There are five major *nitrogenous bases:* adenine, guanine, uracil, uracil, thymine and cytosine. The first two are purines - their molecules consist of two rings, one containing five members, the other six. The next three are pyrimidines and have a single five-membered ring of thymidyl thymidine nucleotide. The names of the nucleotides are derived from the names of the corresponding nitrogenous bases; both are denoted by capital letters: adenine - adenosine (A), guanine - guanosine (G), cytosine - cytidine (C), thymine - thymidine (T), uracil - uridine (U) (Fig. 17).

Sugar, a constituent of a nucleotide, contains five carbon atoms, i.e. it is a pentose, which can be present in one of two forms*: ribose and deoxyribose.* The difference between the two is that the hydrogen atom at the second carbon atom of deoxyribose in ribose is replaced by a hydroxyl group (-OH). The sugar is attached to one of the bases by a glycosidic bond connecting the 1st carbon atom of pentose to the 1st nitrogen atom of pyrimidine derivatives or to the 9th nitrogen atom of purine derivatives.

Depending on the form of pentose, two types of nucleic acids are distinguished: *deoxyribonucleic acid (DNA) and ribonucleic acid (RNA).*

ribonucleic acid (RNA). Nucleic acids are acids because their molecule contains a phosphoric acid residue (-HPO).3

The number of nucleotides in a nucleic acid molecule varies from 80 in transport RNA molecules to several tens of thousands in DNA.

DNA is a double-stranded helix twisted around its own axis. In a polynucleotide chain, neighbouring nucleotides are linked by covalent bonds. Which are formed between the phosphate group of one nucleotide and the 3' - alcoholic pentose group of another. Such bonds are called phosphodiester bonds *(phosphate-sugar-phosphate-sugar*, etc.). The phosphate group forms a bridge between the 3'-carbon of one pentose cycle and the5'-carbon of the next.

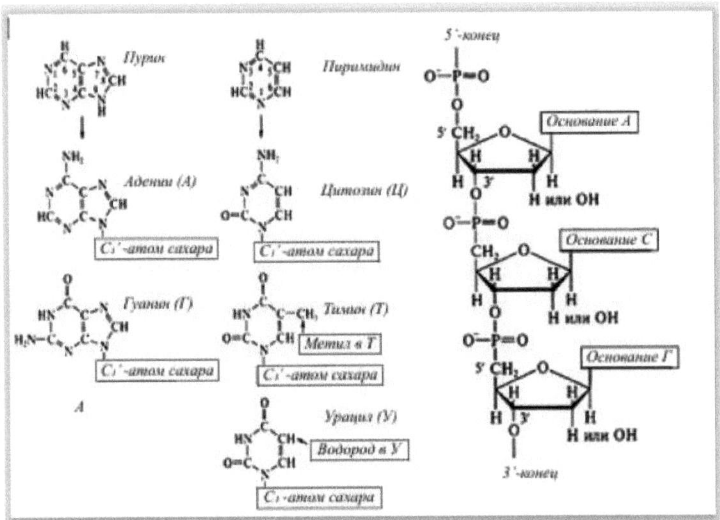

Figure 17: Structure of bases. A- purine derivatives.

Figure 18: Scheme of nucleic acid backbone formation.

B- pyrimidine derivatives.

The backbone of DNA chains is thus formed by sucrose phosphate residues (Figure 18).

The polynucleotide chain of DNA is twisted in a helix, resembling a spiral staircase, and is connected to its complementary chain by hydrogen bonds formed between adenine and thymine (two bonds) and guanine and cytosine (three bonds).

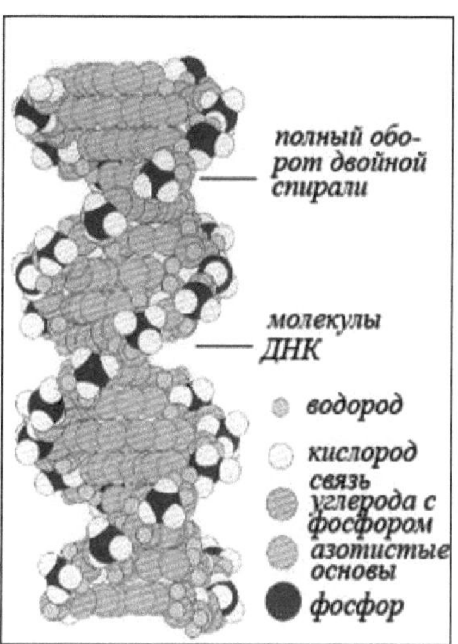

Figure 19: Structure of the DNA molecule.

The nucleotides A and T, G and CD are called *complementary*. As a result, in any organism, the number of adenyl nucleotides equals the number of thymidyl nucleotides, and the number of guanyl nucleotides equals the number of cytidyl nucleotides.

This regularity was named "E. Chargaff's rule". Due to this property, the sequence of nucleotides in one chain determines their sequence in another chain. The chains in a DNA molecule are oppositely directed, i.e. if one chain has a direction from 3' and end to 5' - end, then in another chain 3' - end corresponds to 5' - end and vice versa. This property of DNA bispiral is called *antiparallelism*.

The double-stranded model of the DNA molecule was first proposed in 1953 by the American scientist J.Watson and the Englishman F.Crick. They combined E. Chargaff's data on the ratio of purine and pyrimidine bases of DNA molecules and the results of X-ray structural analysis obtained by M. Wilkins and R. Franklin (Fig. 19).

J. Watson, F. Crick and M. Wilkins were awarded the Nobel Prize in 1962 for the development of the double helix model of the DNA molecule. DNA is the largest biological molecule. Their length ranges from 0.25 mm in some bacteria to 40 mm in humans, which is much larger than the largest protein molecule, which in unfolded form reaches no more than 100 - 200 nm. The mass of a DNA molecule is $6\text{-}10^{12}$ g.

The diameter of the DNA molecule is 2 nm, the helix pitch is 3.4 nm; each turn of the helix contains 10 nucleotide pairs. The helical structure is supported by numerous bonds between complementary nitrogenous bases and hydrophobic interactions.

DNA molecules of eukaryotic organisms are linear. In contrast, in prokaryotes, DNA is closed in a ring and has neither 3'- nor 5'-ends. Like proteins, DNA can undergo *denaturation*, called melting, when conditions change. On gradual return to normal conditions, DNA renaturates.

The function of DNA is to store, transmit and reproduce genetic information over generations. The DNA of any cell contains information about all proteins of a given organism, about which proteins, in what sequence and in what quantity will be synthesised.

The chain containing information about the protein structure (in the 5'3' direction) is called the sense chain, and the complementary chain is called the antisense chain. The antisense strand is of great importance in stabilising the structure of the DNA double helix and is involved in the processes of *replication* and repair of damaged DNA. DNA molecules are giant polymers. The units of measurement of molecule length are: nucleotide pairs *(bp),* thousands of nucleotide pairs - *kilobases (kb),* millions of base pairs - *megabases (mb) (*Fig. 20).

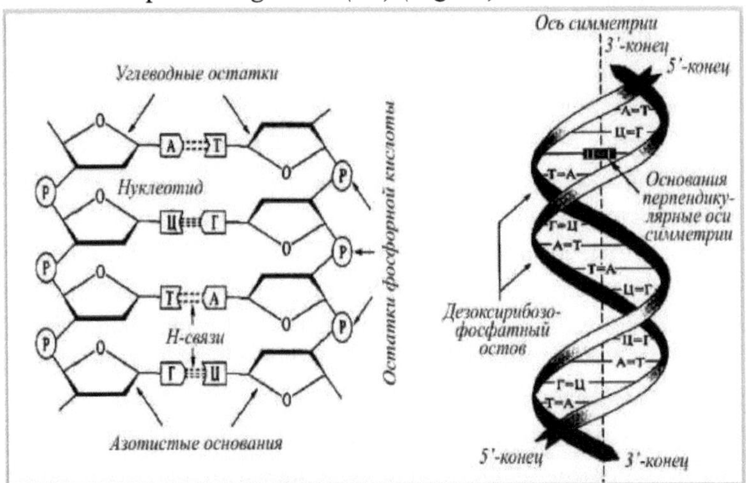

Figure 20: Chain complementarity and schematic of the DNA molecule.

In humans, the haploid set contains 3.2×10^9 nucleotide pairs, or 3.2 billion base pairs. Almost all of the cell's DNA is contained in the nucleus in the form of 46 tightly packed, super-twisted structures - chromosomes - due to interactions with nuclear proteins. A relatively small part of DNA (about

5%) is localised in mitochondria.

RNA. The structure of RNA molecules is similar in many respects to the structure of DNA molecules. However, there are a number of significant differences. In the RNA molecule, instead of deoxyribose, the nucleotides include ribose. Instead of thymidyl nucleotide (T) there is uridine (U). The main difference from DNA is that the RNA molecule is a single strand. However, its nucleotides can form hydrogen bonds between themselves (e.g. in tRNA, rRNA molecules), but in this case it is an intrachain connection of complementary nucleotides.

RNA strands are much shorter than DNA.

Types of RNA. There are several types of RNA in the cell, which differ in molecule size, structure, location in the cell, and function.

Informational (matrix) RNA - mRNA - is the most heterogeneous in size and structure. mRNA is an unclosed polynucleotide chain. It is synthesised in the nucleus with the participation of the RNA polymerase enzyme according to the principle of complementarity to the DNA region responsible for the synthesis of a certain protein. RNA fulfils the most important function in the cell. mRNA serves as a matrix for protein synthesis, transferring information about their structure from DNA molecules. Each protein in the cell is encoded by an mRNA specific to it.

Ribosomal RNA - rRNA. These are single-stranded nucleic acids that, in complex with proteins, form ribosomes - organoids where protein synthesis takes place. Information about the structure of rRNA is encoded in the DNA regions located in the secondary strand of chromosomes. rRNA accounts for 80% of all RNA in the cell, since cells contain a large number of ribosomes. rRNAs have a complex secondary and tertiary structure, forming loops at complementary sites, which leads to self-organisation of these molecules into a complexly shaped body.

Ribosomes are composed of 3 types of rRNA - in prokaryote and 4 types of rRNA - in eukaryote.

Transport (transfer) RNA - tRNA. A tRNA molecule consists of 80 nucleotides on average. The content of tRNA in the cell is about 15% of all RNA. The function of tRNA is to transport amino acids to the site of protein synthesis. The number of different types of tRNAs in the cell is small (about 40). All of them have a similar spatial organisation.

Due to intrachain hydrogen bonds, the tRNA molecule acquires a characteristic secondary structure called a *cloverleaf* (Figure 21).

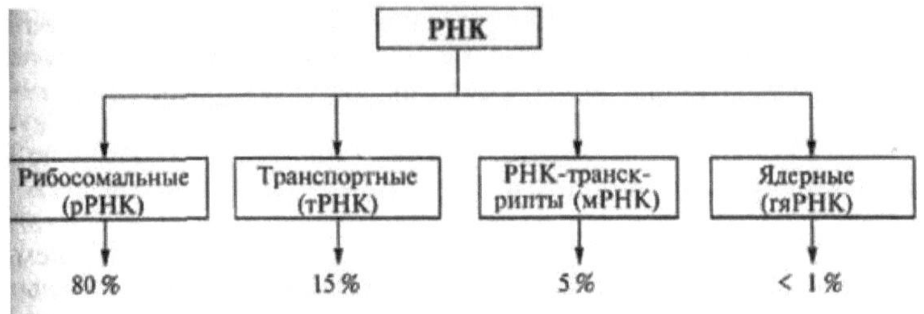

Figure 21: Ratio of RNA species in the cell.

DNA doubling. DNA molecules have a remarkable property that is not inherent in any other known molecule - the ability to double. With the help of special enzymes, the hydrogen bonds that bind DNA strands are broken, the strands diverge, and to each nucleotide of each of these strands are sequentially attached complementary nucleotides. The separated strands of the original (parent) DNA molecule are matrix strands - they set the order of nucleotides in the newly synthesised chain.

As a result of the action of a complex set of enzymes, nucleotides are joined together. New strands are formed

DNA complementary to each of the divergent strands (Figure 22).

Thus, doubling creates two DNA double helixes (daughter molecules), each with one strand derived from the parent molecule and one strand synthesised again.

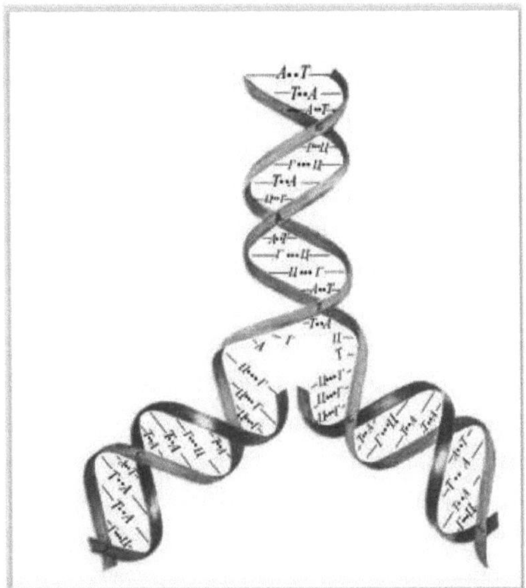

Figure 22: Schematic of DNA doubling.

The process of nucleic acid replication depends entirely on the work of a number of enzymes. At least four groups of enzymes have been found to be involved in this process: *DNA polymerases, RNA polymerases, endonucleases* and *DNA ligases.*

1. The enzymes that carry out DNA synthesis *are* called DNA polymerases.
2. RNA polymerase is the enzyme that carries out RNA transcription.
3. Endonuclease is an enzyme that cuts the double-stranded DNA molecule at sites corresponding to sequences of 4-12 nucleotides.
4. DNA ligases are enzymes that catalyse the formation of a phosphodiester bond between the Z'- and 5'-ends of DNA fragments.

The daughter DNA molecules are not different from each other or from the parent molecule. When a cell divides, the daughter DNA molecules disperse into the two resulting cells, each of which will have the same information that was contained in the mother cell. Since genes are sections of DNA molecules, the two daughter cells that form during cell division have the same genes.

A random error in a gene of a germ cell will be reproduced in the genes of millions of its descendants. This is why all the red blood cells of a sickle cell anaemia patient have the same ***"tainted"*** haemoglobin. Children with anaemia get the "tainted" gene from their parents through their germ cells.

2.3. GENES AND THEIR STRUCTURE

The elementary unit of heredity is a ***gene.*** According to modern concepts, a gene is a section of the genomic DNA molecule characterised by a sequence of nucleotides specific to it, representing a unit of function different from that of other genes, and capable of change by mutation.

A gene is a section of a DNA molecule. It is discrete, as it consists of nucleotides connected in sequence. This is its most accurate characteristic, which makes it possible to identify a given gene, no matter where it is located. Changes in the molecular structure of the DNA of genes, i.e. changes in the nucleic acid of which they are composed, leads to the appearance of new forms of genetic information, new molecular structures in the material structure of heredity. Such changes (mutations) can occur at any point within a gene. But in functional terms, the gene is an integral unit: any change of nucleotides in the gene or loss of its part either completely inactivates it or changes the genetic information embedded in it.

Exon - intronic organisation of a gene. The human gene has a coding part *(exon)* with a total length of several thousand base pairs. However, the total length of the gene is much longer, because in addition to exons, the gene includes *introns* (non-coding part) and *flanking sequences* located before (from the 5'-end) and after (from the Z'-end) the coding part (Fig. 23). The coding part of most genes is within 1-2 thousand base pairs, which corresponds to a protein product of 300-1000 amino acid residues.

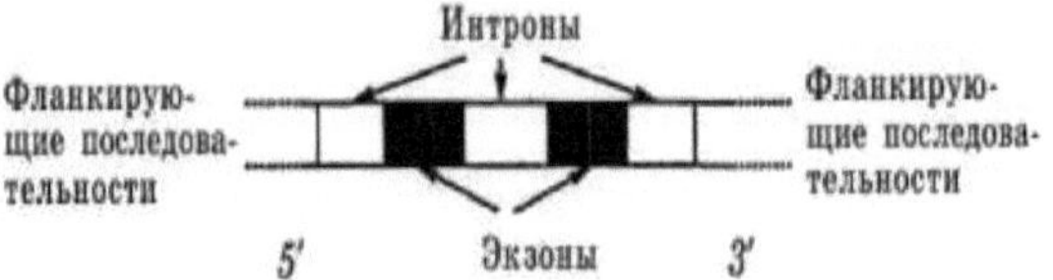

Figure 23: Organisation of a gene.

In most genes, the coding part is divided into several exons, between which non-coding regions, introns, are located. The intergenic regions of DNA are called *spacers*. Spacers consist of repetitive DNA sequences of various types and unique non-transcribed sequences that are not genes. Their function is not known.

A DNA molecule may contain many genes. According to modern estimates, humans have about 30-40 thousand genes, each of which fulfils a specific function - encodes a certain polypeptide or RNA molecules.

2.4. THE GENETIC CODE. TRANSCRIPTION. PROTEIN SYNTHESIS IN THE CELL

The process of iRNA formation. Ribosomes, the sites of protein synthesis, receive from the nucleus an information-carrying intermediary capable of passing through the pores of the nuclear envelope. This intermediary is information RNA (iRNA). It is a single-stranded molecule complementary to one strand of the DNA molecule. A special enzyme - polymerase, moving along DNA, selects nucleotides according to the principle of complementarity and joins them into a single chain.

The process of iRNA formation is called *transcription* (from Latin *"transcription"* - rewriting). If the DNA strand contains thymine, polymerase includes adenine in the iRNA chain, if guanine includes cytosine, if adenine includes uracil (RNA does not include thymine).

The length of each iRNA molecule is hundreds of times shorter than DNA. In prokaryotes, such a group of genes is called an *operon*. In prokaryotes, such a group of genes is called an *operon*.

At the beginning of each group of genes there is a kind of landing pad for polymerase, called a *promoter*. This is a specific sequence of DNA nucleotides that the enzyme "recognises" due to chemical affinity. Only after joining the promoter, the polymerase is able to start synthesising iRNA. At the end of a group of genes, the enzyme encounters a signal (in the form of a specific sequence of nucleotides) that signifies the end of rewriting. The finished iRNA departs from the DNA, leaves the nucleus and goes to the site of protein synthesis, the ribosome, located in the cytoplasm of the cell. In the cell, genetic information is transmitted through transcription from DNA to protein:

$$\text{DNA} \rightarrow \text{iRNA} \rightarrow \text{protein.}$$

Proteins, or proteins, are large polymeric molecules built from monomeric amino acid links that are linked together. Proteins are made up of twenty different amino acids. All amino acids share a common plan of structure. The obligatory elements are: an amino group (*-Nil2*) and a carboxyl group (-COOH) bonded to a central carbon atom. A hydrogen atom (-H) and a radical (side group, denoted by the symbol R) are also linked to it.

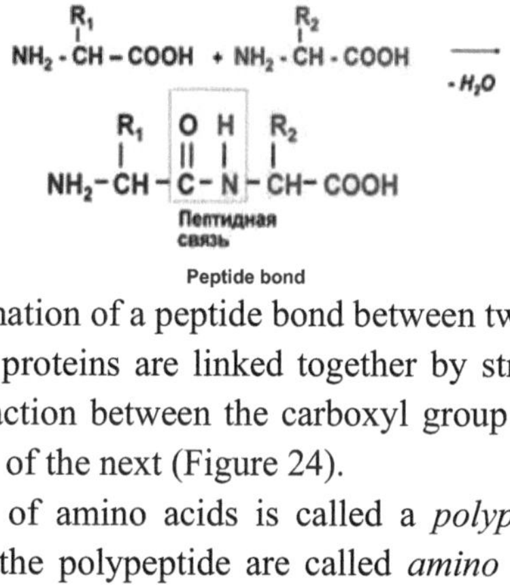

$$NH_2-\underset{|}{\overset{R_1}{CH}}-COOH + NH_2-\overset{R_2}{CH}-COOH \xrightarrow[-H_2O]{} NH_2-\overset{R_1}{CH}-\overset{O}{\overset{\|}{C}}-\overset{H}{\overset{|}{N}}-\overset{R_2}{CH}-COOH$$

Пептидная связь

Peptide bond

Figure 24: Formation of a peptide bond between two amino acids.

The amino acids in proteins are linked together by strong *peptide bonds* formed by the interaction between the carboxyl group of one amino acid and the amino group of the next (Figure 24).

The resulting chain of amino acids is called a *polypeptide.* The amino acids that make up the polypeptide are called *amino acid residues.* The sequence of amino acid residues is called the primary structure of the protein. The terms *"secondary" and "tertiary"* structure refer to the different levels of organisation of this linear sequence. Quaternary structure is protein complexes formed by the interaction of different polypeptide chains (Fig. 25).

Genetic code and its properties. The genetic information contained in DNA and in iRNA is contained in the sequence of nucleotides in the molecules. How does iRNA encode (encrypt) the primary structure of proteins, i.e. the order of amino acids in them. The essence of the code is that the sequence of nucleotides in iRNA determines the sequence of amino acids in proteins. This ***code*** is called the *genetic* ***code,*** *and* its deciphering is one of the great achievements of science.

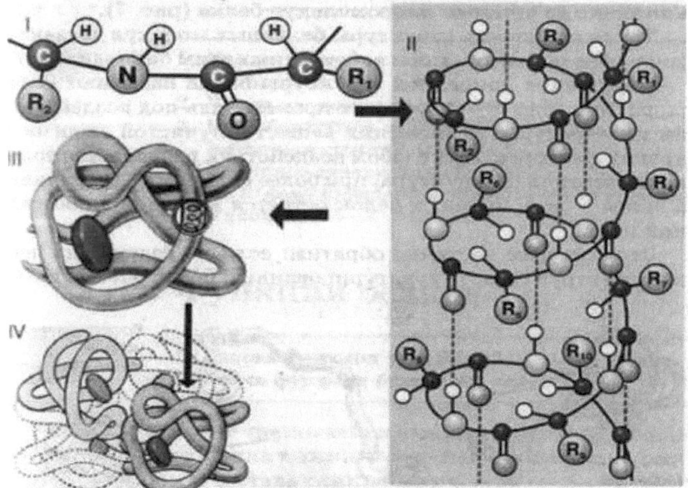

Fig. 25. Structural levels of protein molecules organisation.

The carrier of genetic information is DNA, but since iRNA, a copy of one of the DNA strands, is directly involved in protein synthesis, the genetic code is written in the "language" of RNA.

The code is triplet. RNA contains 4 nucleotides: A, G, C, U. If we tried to designate one amino acid with one nucleotide, we could encode only 4 amino acids, whereas there are 20 amino acids, all of which are used in protein synthesis. A two-letter code would allow us to code 16 amino acids (16 different combinations can be made of 4 nucleotides, each with 2 nucleotides).

In nature, there is a three-letter, or triplet, code. This means that each of the 20 amino acids is encrypted by a sequence of 3 nucleotides, i.e. a triplet, which is called a *codon.* From 4 nucleotides, 64 different combinations of 3 nucleotides each can be created (4^3 =64). This is more than enough to encode 20 amino acids and it would seem that 44 triplets are superfluous. However, this is not the case. Almost *every amino acid is encoded by more than one codon* (from 2 to 6). This can be seen from the table of the genetic code. Properties of the genetic code.

Table 2.

Genetic code table

Amino acid	Coding triplets - codons
Alanine	HZU herculeanGCA GTF

Arginine	TSU	tsgc	CGA	TSG	HAHAAGG
Asparagine	AAU	AAC			
Asparagine acid	GAU	GAC			
Valine	GUU	GUTS	SUA	GUG.	
Histidine	CAU	CAC			
Glycine	GSU	HGC	GHA	YYYYY.	
Glutamine			CAA	CAG	
Glutamic acid			GAA	GAG	
Isoleucine	AUU	ATC	AUA.		
Leucine	CUU	MCC	CUA	TSUG	UUAUUH
Lysine			AAA	AAG	
Methionine				AUG	
Proline	CCC	tsatz	TZCA	CTF	
Cerin	UCU	BYGCA	UCA	DRM	ASUAGC
Tyrosine	WOW.	UAC			
Threonine	ACU	ACC	ACA	ADC	
Tryptophan				UGH	
Phenylalanine	UUU	ATC			
Cysteine	USU	UGC			
Punctuation marks			UGA	UAS	WAA

1. The genetic code is triplet. Each amino acid is encoded by a group of three nucleotides (nucleotide triplet) (Table 2).

2. The outgrowth of the genetic code. One amino acid can be encoded not by one, but by several specific triplets of nucleotides.

3. Unambiguity of the genetic code. Each codon corresponds to only one amino acid, i.e. a triplet encrypts only one amino acid.

4. Non-overlap of the genetic code. The process of reading the genetic code does not allow the possibility of overlapping codons. Having started at a certain codon, reading of the following codons proceeds without skips, i.e. there are no punctuation marks inside the gene. For example, if one or two nucleotides fall out of the chain, the readout produces a protein that has nothing in common with the protein encoded by the normal gene.

5. Universality of the genetic code. Genetic information for all organisms with different levels of organisation (from a daisy to a human) is encoded in the same way.

6. Linearity of the genetic code. Codons are read sequentially in the direction of the encoded record from 5'-end to Z'-end.

Protein biosynthesis. Information RNA, which carries information about the primary structure of protein molecules, is synthesised in the nucleus. After passing through the pores of the nuclear envelope, iRNA is directed to ribosomes, where the genetic information is decoded, i.e. translated from the "language" of nucleotides to the "language" of amino acids.

The amino acids from which proteins are synthesised are delivered to ribosomes by special RNAs called *transport* RNAs *(tRNAs).* There are as many different types of tRNAs in the cell as there are types of codons that encode amino acids. At the top of each tRNA "sheet" there is a sequence of three nucleotides complementary to the nucleotides of the codon in the iRNA.

This sequence of nucleotides in the tRNA structure is called an *anticodon.* A special enzyme "recognises" the anticodon and attaches to the "leaf petiole" of the tRNA not any, but a certain, "own" amino acid. This is the *first step of* protein *synthesis*. In order for an amino acid to be incorporated into the polypeptide chain of a protein, it must detach from the tRNA. In the *second step of synthesis, tRNA* acts as a translator from the "language" of nucleotides to the "language" of amino acids.

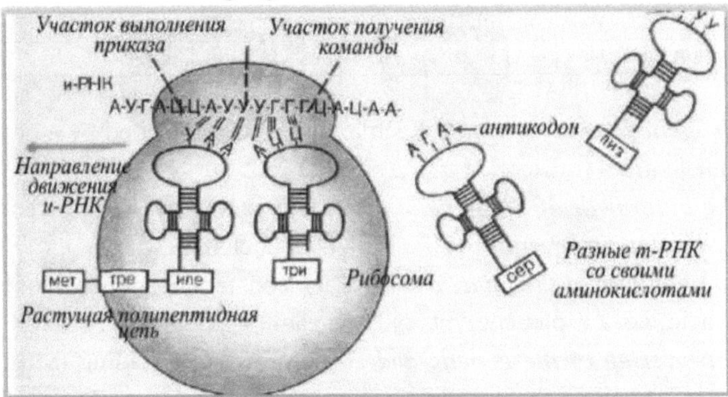

Figure 26: Schematic of protein biosynthesis.

This translation takes place on the ribosome. There are two sites in it: at one tRNA receives a command from iRNA - the anticodon recognises the codon, at the other the order is executed - the amino acid is detached from tRNA (Fig. 26).

The third step in protein ***synthesis*** is that the enzyme synthetase attaches the amino acid detached from the tRNA to the growing polypeptide chain. The informative RNA slides continuously across the ribosome, each triplet first entering the first site, where it is recognised by the tRNA anticodon, then the second site. This is where the tRNA with the amino acid attached to it goes, and here the amino acids are detached from the tRNA and joined together in the sequence in which the triplets follow one after the other.

When one of the three triplets, which are punctuation marks between genes, is found on the ribosome at the first site, it means that protein synthesis is complete. The finished polypeptide chain moves away from the ribosome. The process of synthesising a protein molecule requires a large expenditure of energy. In addition, the energy of several ATP molecules is needed to move the iRNA across the ribosome. To increase protein production, the iRNA often simultaneously passes through not one, but several ribosomes in series. Such a structure united by a single molecule of iRNA is called a ***polysome.*** On each ribosome, several molecules of identical proteins are synthesised sequentially in this bead-like conveyor belt. Amino acids are interruptlessly delivered to the ribosomes by tRNA. After giving up an amino acid, the tRNA molecule immediately combines with another amino acid of the same type. The high coherence of all

The "plant services" of protein production allow synthesising molecules consisting of hundreds of amino acids within a few minutes. Protein synthesis on ribosomes is called *translation* (from Latin, *"translatio"* - transfer).

Control Questions and Assignments:

1. What nucleic acids do you know, how are they different?
2. What is a DNA molecule?
3. What is the rule of complementarity?
4. List the types of RNAs and their functions.
5. What is DNA replication.
6. Give a definition of the genetic code.
7. What is an exon and what is an intron?
8. How is genetic information decoded?
9. List the properties of the genetic code.
10. Does the genetic code differ between different species of living things?

TEST-2.

1. DNA replication is....

a) process of DNA molecule doubling; b) reading process

(c) The process of transmitting hereditary information;

e) synthesis of RNA on a DNA matrix.

2. The exchange of sites between homologous chromatids during meiosis is called ... .

a) duplication; b) conjugation;

c) crossing-over; e) gene fusion.

3. Identify the correct statements:

1) i-RNA, consisting of 270 nucleotides, is involved in the synthesis of a protein containing 89 peptide bonds;

2) DNA, consisting of 210 nucleotides, is involved in the synthesis of a protein consisting of70 amino acids;

3) An i-RNA containing 120 ribose molecules forms a polypeptide with 40 peptide bonds;

4) from DNA, which has 358 phosphodiester nucleotides, to form i-RNA, which contains 180 molecules of ribose.

A) 2,4 B) 1,4 C) 1,3 E) 2,3

4. Identify the correct statements:

1) i-RNA, consisting of 132 nucleotides, is involved in the synthesis of a protein containing 44 peptide bonds;

2) 40 amino acids are formed from T-DNA, which has 240 nucleotides;

3) An i-RNA containing 210 ribose molecules forms a polypeptide with 69 peptide bonds;

4) from DNA, which has 178 nucleotides, to form i-RNA, which contains 90 molecules of ribose.

A)2,3 B)2,4 C)1,3D)1,4

5. An i-RNA molecule contains 80 uracil nucleotides, which make up 40% of the total number of nucleotides. Determine the phosphodiester bonds in the DNA with which this RNA is synthesised (the distance between DNA nucleotides is 0.34 nm).

A) 399 B) 198 C) 199D) 398

CHALLENGE-2.

1. One of the chains of a DNA molecule has the following nucleotide order:

AAGGCTCTTTAGGTAGGTAGGTAGTAGTAGTAGTAGTAGT.

a) . Determine the sequence of nucleotides in the complementary chain.

б) . Determine the codon sequence of the iRNA synthesised on the complementary strand.

в) . Determine the sequence of amino acids in the polypeptide encoded in the complementary chain.

2. A single strand of DNA is given. TTCGAGATCGTCGTCA.

Make an example diagram and explain the principle of complementarity of nitrogenous bases of DNA and RNA molecules.

3. Considering that the average molecular mass of an amino acid is about 110 and that of a nucleotide is about 300, determine which is heavier: the protein or the gene?

4. The nucleic acid of a phage has a molecular mass of about 107. How many proteins, approximately, are encoded in it, assuming that a typical protein consists of 400 monomers on average and the molecular mass of a nucleotide is about 300?

5. In a person with cystinuria (a higher than normal number of amino acids in the urine), the amino acids that correspond to the following triplets of informational RNA are excreted in the urine: UTSU, UGU, GTSU, GGU, GGU, TSAA, AGA, AAA. In a healthy person, alanine, serine, glutamic acid and glycine are found in the urine.

Which amino acid excretion in urine is characteristic of patients with cystinuria?

CHAPTER III

THE BASICS OF GENETICS.

3.1. LAWS OF INHERITANCE

History of the development of genetics. The fact that organisms transmit traits and properties to their offspring has long been intuitively known. This knowledge was used in agriculture, when a peasant, wishing to get more grain, tried to leave the largest seeds from the most productive plants for sowing. Naturally, people could not understand the regularities of inheritance of traits for a long time. The first attempts to explain the fact that children usually resemble their parents were made by Hippocrates, the great scientist and physician of Ancient Greece. Such reports are found in the works of Aristotle, Plato and other ancient Greek physicians, and philosophers. The fact that they not only described cases of inheritance of certain traits, but also offered theoretical explanations and even measures to improve human nature is remarkable. After the Renaissance, interest in human nature increased. Thus, the work of the Spanish physician Mercado (1605) contains a statement that both parents, not only the father, determine what the future child will be like. Already in the XVIII - early XIX centuries there were works that gave a correct assessment of hereditary diseases and the nature of their transmission. For example, in 1752 in the work of Maupertuis reported on a family with polydactyly in four generations. Observations of this family allowed the author to conclude that this malformation was equally transmitted by both father and mother, and calculations showed that the high frequency of this pathology could not be explained by chance alone. Among the works of this period, special attention should be paid to "A Treatise on the Presumed Hereditary Properties of Disease" by the English physician and researcher Adams, in which he drew a number of remarkable conclusions: the existence of hereditary (dominant) and familial (recessive) factors. Another important conclusion from his work is that diseases that are identical in their clinical manifestations may have different genetic natures. In the works of Professor of Medicine Nasse (1820), the most important signs of haemophilia inheritance were identified.

However, in the works of most researchers of the 19th century, true factors and erroneous ideas about heredity were mixed up. This was a typical state of affairs in genetics at the "pre-scientific" stage of its development. Among the researchers of the 19th century, F. Galton should be particularly emphasised, who justified the twin, clinical and 62 genealogical and biometric methods for studying human heredity. In Russia in the 19th century, heredity was considered by doctors as an etiological and pathogenetic factor; many hereditary diseases were known. Genealogical method was included in anamnesis.

However, the lack of correct ideas about the patterns of inheritance of traits led to confusion of concepts and contradictory conclusions. The scientific period of genetics began in 1900, when Mendel's laws were rediscovered.

H.Mendel's experiments and the conclusions drawn from them laid down the concept of the gene, which is formulated by analysing certain crosses. When H.Mendel conducted his experiments, nothing was known about possible material carriers of genetic information in germ cells. However, in the following decades until the end of the 19th century, chromosomes were discovered and mitosis and meiosis were investigated. Soon after the rediscovery of Mendel's laws, when comparing the Mendelian cleavage of traits and the distribution of chromosomes in meiosis, it was finally concluded that it was the chromosomes that were the carriers of genetic information. The birth of genetics was the beginning of a new scientific period of development, which successfully continues to this day, shedding new light on the hidden mystery of human nature.

Hybridological method. The main method, which H. Mendel developed and put in the basis of his experiments, is called the *hybridological method.* Its essence consists in crossing organisms that differ from each other in one or several features. Since the offspring from such crosses are called *hybrids*, the method is called hybridological.

One of the peculiarities of H. Mendel's method was that he used *pure lines* for experiments, i.e. plants, in the offspring of which no diversity in the studied trait was observed during self-pollination. A trait is usually understood as any feature of an organism, i.e. any individual quality, by which two individuals can be distinguished. For example, flower colour white and purple, plant maturation rate precocity and late maturity, flower height high and low. In humans, resistance or susceptibility to disease, etc.

The totality of all traits of an organism, starting from external and ending with features of structure and functioning of cells and organs, is called *phenotype.* This term can also be used in relation to one of the alternative (mutually exclusive, contrasting) traits.

The development of all hereditary traits and properties of an organism is determined by the *genotype,* i.e. the totality of genes and their cytoplasmic carriers interacting with each other. The concepts of *"genotype"* and *"phenotype" are* very important in genetics. Phenotype is formed under the influence of genotype and environmental conditions. An equally important feature of the method is the accurate quantitative accounting of each pair of alternative traits in a series of generations.

Mathematical processing of experimental data allowed G.Mendel to establish quantitative regularities in the transmission of the studied traits. It was very important that H. Mendel in his experiments followed an analytical way: he observed the inheritance of diverse traits not at once in the totality, but only one pair (or a small number of pairs) of alternative traits. The hybridological method is also the basis of modern genetics.

The basic laws of H. Mendel. H.Mendel, based on the results of his experiments on crossbreeding different varieties of peas, formulated regularities known nowadays as Mendel's laws.

H.Mendel's first law (the law of uniformity of hybrids of the first generation or the law of dominance): when homozygous parental forms with opposite traits are crossed in the first generation of offspring (F1), all individuals are homotypic *(uniform)* in genotype and phenotype. The trait that appeared in F1 was called *dominant*, and the trait of the second parental form, which was suppressed, was called *recessive.*

Let us refer to the diagram on which symbols record the results of the experiment on monohybrid crossing (crossing of parental forms differing only in one trait).

P. ♀AA x ♂aa
G. A a

F 1Aa - 100% by phenotype: all dominant

by genotype: all heterozygous.

Homozygous and heterozygous individuals. H.Mendel for the first time established the fact that plants similar in appearance can differ sharply in hereditary properties. Individuals that do not give cleavage in the next generation, received the

homozygous (from Greek *"homos"* - equal, *"zygote"* - fertilised egg). Individuals that show cleavage in their offspring are called *heterozygous* (from Greek *"heteros"* - other).

H.Mendel's second law (law of cleavage): when two heterozygous individuals, analysed by one pair of alternative traits, are crossed, in the offspring there is a cleavage in phenotype in the ratio of 3:1, in genotype in the ratio of 1:2:1.

Let's refer to the diagram:

P. ♀ **Aa x** ♂**Aa**
G. **A, a** **A, a**
F_1 AA; Aa; Aa; aa.
3 yellow 1 green (by phenotype)

1AA : 2AA : 1aa (pogenotype).

Conclusion:

1. Individual traits of organisms do not disappear in crossbreeding, but are retained in the offspring.
2. Each gamete receives only one gene from a given allele pair, and the number of gametes carrying carved alleles of the same gene is the same.
3. Male and female gametes carrying different alleles of the same gene are combined randomly at fertilisation.

Note: Symbols P, Fi, F2, etc. denote parental, first and second generations, respectively. Symbol X - crossing, $ - female sex (Venus mirror), **<$** - male sex (Mars shield and spear) and G - gametes.

The principle of gamete purity. The rule of gamete purity established by Mendel indicates the discreteness of a gene, the non-mixing of alleles with each other and with other genes.

In monohybrid crosses, in the case of dominance in heterozygous hybrids (Aa) of the first generation, only the dominant allele (A) is manifested; the recessive allele (a) is not lost or mixed with the dominant allele. In the second generation, both recessive and dominant alleles can be manifested in their "pure" form, i.e. in the homozygous state. In this case, the hereditary factors not only do not mix, but also do not undergo changes after being together in the hybrid organism.

As a result, the gametes formed by such a heterozygote are "pure" in the sense that gamete (A) is "pure" and contains nothing from allele (a); gamete (a) is "pure" from allele (A).

The cytological basis of gamete purity (allele discreteness) consists in their localisation in different chromosomes of each homologous pair, and gene discreteness - in their localisation in different loci of chromosomes.

Analysing crossbreeding. It is not always possible to determine the genotype of an individual from its phenotype. In analytical crossbreeding, the individual whose genotype is to be determined is crossed with individuals homozygous for the recessive gene, i.e. having the genotype (aa).

Let's look at analytical crossbreeding with an example:

1. **P.**	♀AA x ♂ aa		**2. P.**	♀Aa x ♂aa	
G.	A	a	G.	A, a	a
F_1.		Aa	F_1.	1Aa :	laa
		100%		50% :	50%.

The examples show that individuals homozygous for the dominant gene do not cleave in F1, while heterozygous individuals crossed with a homozygous individual give cleavage already in F1.

Incomplete dominance or intermediate inheritance is observed when the phenotype of a heterozygous hybrid differs from the phenotype of both parental forms, i.e. the expression of the trait is intermediate, with a greater or lesser bias towards one or the other parent. The mechanism of this phenomenon is that the recessive allele is inactive. And the degree of activity of the dominant allele is insufficient to ensure the desired level of appearance of the trait of the dominant parental homozygote. For example, when a plant Night Beauty with white flowers is crossed with a plant that has red flowers, all F 1 hybrids have pink flowers.

P. ♀AA x ♂aa

hair dryer: red white

F_1. Aa

Pink

P. ♀Aa x ♂Aa

hair dryer: pink pink.

F_1. AA; Aa; Aa; aa.

hair dryer: red pink white

gen: 1AA : 2aa : laa.

Incomplete dominance has turned out to be a widespread phenomenon. It is observed in the inheritance of curly hair in humans, cattle colouring, plumage colouring in chickens, and many other morphological and physiological traits in humans.

The third law of H. Mendel (the law of independent cleavage): each pair of traits cleaves independ***ently*** of other pairs of traits. This law is valid only for genes located either in different chromosomes or in one chromosome but far enough from each other. Mendel's exact cleavage can be expected only when the analysed offspring is large enough. Let us consider H. Mendel's experiment, in which he studied independent inheritance of traits in peas.

When crossing homozygous individuals differing in two or more pairs of alternative traits, in the second generation (F_2) in F1 *inbreeding*, independent combination of traits is observed, resulting in hybrid forms bearing traits in combinations not peculiar to the parental and progenitor individuals. For example,

P. ♀AABB x ♂aaвв **G. AB aв** **F_1 AaBв - 100%**	A- yellow colour; a-green B- smooth shape; c - wrinkled shape.

All individuals are heterozygous for the phenotype and with dominant traits exhibited in the phenotype. Inbreeding F 1:

P. $ AaBv x $ AaBv

G. AB; Av; av; aV; av; av; av; av; av;

gametes ♂ ♀	AB	Av	aB	av
AB	AABB	AABW	AABB	AaBv
Av	AABV	Aavv	AaBv	Aavv
aB	AABB	AaBv	aaBB	aaBv
Av	AaBv	Aavv	aaBv	aavv

When analysing the second generation, it can be seen that 9 genotypes are formed: *AABB, AaBB, AaBB, AaBb, AaBB, aaBB, aaBb, Aabb, Aabb, aabb* and 4 phenotypes: yellow, smooth; green, smooth; yellow, wrinkled; green wrinkled.

In order to shorten the record, similar phenotypes are sometimes labelled by a *phenotypic radical* - this is the part of an organism's genotype that determines its phenotype. For a dihybrid cross, it will be:

$$9\,A\_B\_ : 3\,A\_bb : 3\,aaB\_ : 1\,aabb.$$

Out of 16 possible combinations, in 9 cases 2 dominant traits are realised (AB, i.e. yellow and smooth). In 3 cases, the first trait is dominant, the second recessive (Av, i.e. yellow and wrinkled). In another 3 cases, the first trait is recessive, the second dominant (aB, i.e. green and smooth), and in one case both traits are recessive (Av, green and wrinkled).

Thus, individuals that carry combinations of traits that are not peculiar to the parental forms are manifested - these are yellow, wrinkled peas (Av) and green, smooth (aB). This indicates the independent inheritance of seed shape from seed colour.

If we count separately for each trait (and not in combination with each other), i.e. either by shape or colour, then for each trait the result will be the same as for monohybrid crossing (3:1). If we take into account that in the first generation, when two homozygotes differing in 2 pairs of alternative traits were crossed, a uniform offspring was obtained, then we should conclude that the I and II laws of H. Mendel and the rule of "purity of gametes" are valid for dihybrid crossing as well.

If individuals are analysed for more than two pairs of alternative traits, the number of expected combinations increases. For example, in a trihybrid cross, heterozygotes form 8 types of gametes giving 64 combinations. When counting the phenotypes obtained in this case, the split is observed in the ratio: 27:9:9:9:9:3:3:3:3:1. Solving problems on di- and polyhybrid crosses in many cases can be done without drawing the Pennett grid.

It is important to remember the mathematical patterns in different types of crossbreeding, which are presented in (Table 3).

An obligatory condition for independent combination of traits is the localisation of allelic genes corresponding to them in different (non-homologous) chromosomes. In meiosis, the alleles of alternative traits, because of their localisation in homologous chromosomes, will necessarily end up in different gametes, since the divergence of chromosomes in the anaphase of meiosis 1 proceeds independently. It is quite natural that allele "A" can enter both the gamete where allele "B" will depart and the gamete where allele "B" has entered.

Table 3. Quantitative regularities of gamete formation and hybrid splitting at different types of crossing

Factors taken into account	Type of crossbreeding			
	mono-hybrid	di-hybrid	triple hybrid	poly-hybrid
Number of gamete types produced by the F1 hybrid	2^1	2^2	2^3	2^n
Number of zygotes in the formation of F2	4^1	4^2	4^3	4^n
Number of BF2 phenotypes	2^1	2^2	2^3	2^n
Number of BF 2 genotypes	3^1	3^2	3^3	3^n

Phenotype splitting	$(3+1)^1$	$(3+1)^2$	$(3+1)^3$	$(3+1)^n$
Splitting by genotype	$(1+2+1)^1$	$(1+2+1)^2$	$(1+2+1)^3$	$(1+2+1)^n$

So, the cytological basis of H. Mendel's Law III:

1. Pairing of alleles localised in homologous chromosomes.
2. Independent divergence of homologous chromosomes during meiosis.
3. An independent combination of the two at fertilisation.

3.2. CONDITIONS FOR THE FULFILMENT OF INHERITANCE LAWS

The above-mentioned regularities of trait inheritance are fulfilled only under certain conditions. It is necessary that all types of gametes are formed with equal probability, possess equal viability and participate in fertilisation with equal efficiency, forming all types of zygotes with equal frequency, and zygotes must be characterised by equal viability.

The degree of expression of the trait must also be unchanged. Failure to fulfil at least one of these conditions leads to distorted splits.

For example, if in a monohybrid cross in which there is a split in F_2 *1/4AAA:2/4AA:2/4AA:1/4aa*, there is selective death of zygotes of the AA genotype, then the phenotypic split will look like *2/Zaa:1/Zaa.*

A clear example of this action of genes are hereditary diseases of monogenic nature, i.e. caused by a single gene mutation.

For example, *brachydactyly* (shortening of fingers), *sickle cell anaemia* (a group of pathological conditions defined by the haemoglobin genotypes SS, SC, SD and ST - *thalassaemia*, i.e. genotypes in which at least one of the genes determines the production of sickle cell haemoglobin (HbS).

The exception is persons with AS genotype who are practically healthy. Sickle cell anaemia is characterised by chronic haemolytic anaemia with periodic crises).

It should be noted that even if the above conditions are fulfilled, the actual cleavage does not always correspond exactly to the theoretically calculated one. The point is that the laws of inheritance discovered by Mendel are manifested on a rather large statistical material. For their exact fulfilment, it is necessary to analyse a sample of a certain size.

Thus, the patterns of inheritance are biological in essence, but have a statistical nature of manifestation.

3.3. GENE INTERACTIONS.

3.3.1. ALLELIC GENE INTERACTION

The phenomenon when several genes (alleles) are responsible for one trait is called *gene interaction.* And if they are alleles of the same gene, such interactions are called *allelic*, and in the case of different genes - *non-allelic.*

The following main types of allelic interactions are distinguished: dominance, incomplete dominance and codominance.

Dominance is a type of interaction between two alleles of one gene, in which one of the genes completely excludes the manifestation of the other. As a result, heterozygous organisms phenotypically correspond exactly to the parent homozygous for the dominant alleles. Examples of complete dominance are the dominance of purple colour of pea flowers over white smooth seeds over wrinkled ones; in humans, dark hair over light hair, brown eyes over blue eyes, etc.

However, soon after the secondary discovery of H. Mendel's laws, facts indicating the existence of other forms of intergenic relationships in the genotype system were discovered. Thus, it turned out that domination of some traits over others is a widespread but not universal phenomenon. In some cases, *incomplete dominance* takes place: hybrid F_1 is characterised by a trait intermediate between the parental ones.

Such an example is the appearance of pink coloured lion's zebra flowers when red and white coloured flowers are crossed. In this case, the differences in colouration are due to a pair of allelic genes in which there is no dominance.

Many, perhaps even all, genes in different organisms exist in more than two allelic forms, although a single diploid organism cannot carry more than two alleles.

Multiple alleles were first discovered at the *"white"* locus in Drosophila by T. Morgan and his co-workers. The peculiarity of allelic relationships is that alleles can be arranged in a series in descending order of dominance. Thus, the red-eye gene - the wild (most common in nature) type - will dominate over all other alleles. There are about fifteen of them in total. Each successive member of the allele series will dominate all other members except the previous one.

The existence of multiple alleles itself indicates the relative nature of dominance, as does the fact that they are manifested under specific environmental conditions.

Multiple allelism or codominance - participation of both alleles (paternal and maternal) in determining a trait in a heterozygous individual. In various combinations of genes, both genes are equivalent - they are inherited according to the principle of codominance (not suppressing each other). A vivid and well-studied example of codominance is the inheritance of antigenic human blood groups according to the AVO system.

The ABO blood type (read "a, b, zero") is controlled by a single autosomal gene, that is, a gene located on one of the autosomal (non-sex) chromosomes. The locus of this gene *is* denoted by the Latin letter I (from the word *"isohaemagglutinogen"*), and its three alleles I^o , I^A , I^B are denoted for brevity as A, B, and O. The A and B alleles are codominant with respect to each other, and both are dominant with respect to the O allele. When different alleles are combined, 4 blood types can be formed. The condition where one gene has more than one allelic form is called *multiple allelism.* With homozygosity I^A I^A , red blood cells have only antigen A (blood type A, or II). In homozygosity I^B I^B , red blood cells carry only the B antigen (blood type B, or III). In case of homozygosity I^o I^o the red blood cells are devoid of antigens A and B (blood group O, or I). In the case of heterozygosity I^A I^o or I^B I^o blood type is defined as A(II) or B(III), respectively. In heterozygous individuals with genotype I^A I^B , red blood cells carry both antigens (blood type AB, or IV). The alleles I^A and I^B work in the heterozygote as if independent of each other, which is called *codominance.*

Similarly, in humans, the blood type is determined by the MN system. The alleles controlling the synthesis of two types of proteins (M and N) interact by codominance.

3.3.2. NON-ALLELIC GENE INTERACTION

In the previous section, we considered the patterns of interallelic relationships, i.e., relationships between alleles of the same gene: dominance, incomplete dominance, codominance, and a series of multiple alleles. However, a large number of traits are formed with the participation of several genes, the interaction of which significantly affects the features of the phenotype and leads to deviation from the Mendelian pattern of phenotype splitting.

Several types of interaction between non-allelic genes have been described. It leads to the appearance in the offspring of diheterozygotes of unusual phenotype splitting: 9:3:4; 9:7; 9:6:1; 13:3; 12:3:1; 15:1, i.e.

modification of the general Mendelian formula 9:3:3:1. Cases of interaction between two, three and more non-allelic genes are known. The following main types can be distinguished among them: *complementarity, epistasis, and polymery.*

Complementary or **complementary,** is the interaction of non-allelic dominant genes, resulting in a new trait, which cause the development of a new trait absent in the parents.

For example, crossing two varieties of sweet peas with white flowers produces offspring with purple flowers. If we denote the genotype of one white race by AAVB and the other by AABB, then

P. AAbb x aaBB

white whites

Gametes

Ab aB

F_1: AaBb

AaBv

purple

The first-generation hybrid with two dominant genes (A and B) provided the biochemical basis for the production of the purple pigment anthocyanin, while individually neither gene A nor gene B provided synthesis of this pigment. Anthocyanin synthesis is a complex chain of sequential biochemical reactions controlled by several non-allelic genes, and only in the presence of at least two genes (A-B-) does purple colour develop. In other cases (AaB- and A-B-), the flowers of the plant are white (the sign "-" in the genotype formula means that this place can be occupied by either dominant or recessive allele).

During self-pollination of sweet pea plants from F1 to F_2 , a split into purple- and white-flowered forms was observed in a ratio close to 9:7. Purple flowers were found in 9/16 plants, white flowers in 7/16 plants.

An example of complementary gene interaction in humans is the formation in immunocompetent cells of the body of a specific protein interferon associated with the interaction of two non-allelic genes localised in different chromosomes, or there may be cases when deaf parents give birth to children with normal hearing.

The development of normal hearing is under the genetic control of dozens of different non-allelic genes, the homozygous recessive state of one of which can lead to one of the forms of hereditary deafness. More than 30 such forms are known in humans. If one of the parents is homozygous for the recessive gene aa and the other is homozygous for another recessive gene bb, all their children will be double heterozygotes and, therefore, hearing, since the dominant alleles will complement each other. Thus, a new trait is formed in relation to the parents - normal hearing.

Epistasis (from Greek *epi* - over + *stasis* - obstacle) is a type of gene interaction in which a gene of one allele pair suppresses the manifestations of another. Genes that suppress the action of other genes are called *epistatic, inhibitors* or *suppressors.* The gene that is suppressed is called *a hypostatic gene.*

According to the change in the number and ratio of phenotypic classes of dihybrid cleavage in F_2 several types of epistatic interactions are considered: dominant epistasis (A>B or B>A) with a 12:3:1 cleavage; recessive epistasis (a>B or B>a), which is expressed as a 9:3:4 cleavage, etc.

Epistasis can be compared to complete dominance. In both cases, suppression of one allele by another is observed. However, in epistasis, these are alleles of different genes, while in dominance, they are alleles of one gene. An example of gene interaction by the type of recessive epistasis is the suppression of pigment synthesis in homozygotes for the recessive gene of albinism (aa). Actually, pigment synthesis is controlled by several non-allelic genes, and the albinism gene in the homozygous recessive state prevents the manifestation of these non-allelic genes. Here is another example of recessive epistasis in humans called "Bombay phenotype". It is known that inheritance of ABO blood groups in humans is under the control of one gene (I), which has 3 alleles - I^A , I^B , I^o . In order to realise the information of each allele, the dominant allele H of another gene locus must be present.

If an individual is a recessive homozygote for the H system (i.e. hh), allele 1^B of the ABO system cannot manifest. A person with the genetic constitution of BB and HE must have blood group III. If he or she is simultaneously homozygous for hh, the B allele will not manifest itself in the agglutination reaction, and the person will be recognised as having blood group I.

Polymery (from Greek *polys* - many + *meros* - part) is a type of interaction when the effects of several non-allelic genes determining the same trait are approximately the same. Such traits are called quantitative or polymeric traits. As a rule, the degree of manifestation of polymeric traits depends on the number of dominant genes. The inheritance of polymeric traits was first described by the Swedish geneticist G. Nelson-Ele in 1908. By crossing different forms of wheat (with red and white grains), he observed a cleavage in F2 of the colour trait in the ratio: 15/16 (coloured and '/16 white. Among the coloured grains he observed all transitions - from intensely coloured to weakly coloured.

Analysis of the cleavage features showed that in this case two dominant alleles of two different genes determine the colouration of grains, and combinations of their recessive alleles determine the absence of colouration. Since polymeric genes have unidirectional action, they are usually labelled with the same letters. Thus, the original parental forms had genotypes A1A_1 A2A2 and a1 ai a_2 a_2 . The presence of all four dominant alleles determined the most intense colouring, three dominant alleles (type A 1 A 1 A2A2) - less intense colouring, etc.

An example of polymeric inheritance in humans is the inheritance of skin colouration. In a marriage between an individual of the Negroid race (native African) with black skin and a member of the Caucasoid race with white skin, children are born with intermediate skin colour (mulatto).

Table 4.

Types of non-allelic gene interactions on phenotype.

Type of interaction	Splitting of traits in F_2	Examples
Complementarity is the Interaction of two non-allelic genes leading to a new trait.	9 : 3 : 3 : 1 9 : 6 : 1 9 : 7	Inheritance of plumage colour in parrots. Appearance of disc-shaped fruits in spherical-shaped pumpkins. Inheritance of flower colouration in sweet pea.
Epistasis is a type of interaction between non-allelic genes in which Suppression of the action of an allele of one gene by an allele of another gene occurs.	12 : 3 : 1 13: 3 9 : 3 : 4	**Dominant epistasis.** Breeding by colour in horses. Inheritance of plumage colour in chickens. **Recessive epistasis.** Inheritance of red, yellow-brown and white seed colouration in beans.
Polymergy is an interaction between non-allelic genes in which The manifestation of a trait	1 : 4 : 6 : 4 : 1 (15: 1) 15 : 1	**Cumulative polymerisation.** Inheritance of wheat grain colouration.

depends on the number of dominant genes.		**Non-cumulative polymerisation.** Inheritance of pod shape in shepherd's pouch.

In the marriage of two mulattoes, the offspring can have any skin colour from black to white, because skin pigmentation is caused by the action of three or four non-allelic genes. The effect of each of these genes on skin colouration is about the same.

Polymeric inheritance is characteristic of so-called quantitative traits, such as height, weight, skin colouration, the rate of biochemical reactions, blood pressure, blood sugar, nervous system features, intelligence, and many others that cannot be decomposed into clear phenotypic classes. The greater the number of non-allelic genes controlling the development of a quantitative trait, the less noticeable are the transitions between phenotypic classes.

It is important to remember a few patterns in different types of crosses for non-allelic gene interactions, which are summarised in (Table 4).

3.3.3. PLEIOTROPIC EFFECT OF GENES

Pleiotropic action of a gene is understood as independent or autonomous action of a gene in different organs and tissues, in other words, the influence of one gene on the formation of several traits. A clear example of pleiotropic action of genes are hereditary diseases of monogenic nature, i.e. caused by mutation of one gene, but manifested in different organs or organ systems. Pleiotropic action of genes has different mechanisms, Primary pleiotropy is caused by biochemical mechanisms of action of mutant protein or enzyme - primary products of mutagenic alleles. To illustrate this point, let us give examples.

Mutant alleles of various genes controlling collagen and fibrillin synthesis lead to impaired properties of connective tissue. Since connective tissue is the basis of all organs and tissues, the multiple influence of these mutations on the clinical picture (phenotype) in such inherited connective tissue diseases as, for example, Ehlers-Danlo syndrome and Marfan syndrome, manifested, in particular, by characteristic changes in the bone system, prolapse of the mitral valve of the heart, dilatation of the aortic arch, subluxation of the lens (a consequence of weakness of the cinnamon ligament) is understandable. Another example is multiple lesions 76 neurofibromatosis, where the primary pleiotropic effect of the mutant gene will result in lesions of the nervous and bone systems, skin and visual organs, and other symptoms. Another example of a primary pleiotropic effect of a gene is the characteristic symptoms of an inherited syndrome such as Bardet-Biedl syndrome, which is manifested by a combination of obesity, hexapalatia of the hands and/or feet, underdevelopment of the genitals, mental retardation and characteristic visual impairment in affected individuals.

The multiplicity of organismal lesions may be due to complications of primary pathological processes, between which a relationship can be traced. This is the phenomenon of secondary pleiotropy. For example, in one of the monogenic, autosomal recessively inherited diseases - cystic fibrosis - there is an error in the synthesis of transmembrane protein that provides ion transport in the cells of exocrine glands. Disorders of Na and CI ion transport lead to the formation of thick mucus in the bronchi, the exocrine part of the pancreas or other exocrine glands (sex and sweat glands), which entails secondary inflammatory processes, blockage of excretory ducts, impaired digestion and development of secondary inflammatory processes.

3.3.4. PENETRANCE AND EXPRESSIVITY

The concept of ***penetrance*** refers to the disease as a whole and defines the frequency of phenotype matching a certain genotype. Penetrance can be defined as the frequency of manifestation of a gene in known carriers of the gene. Penetrance can be complete (or 100%) if all carriers of a gene show its clinical (phenotypic) manifestations. If the effect of a gene is not manifested in all its carriers, we speak of incomplete penetrance. In this case, a carrier of a "pathological" gene (even a dominant one) may be clinically healthy. In the case of incomplete penetrance in a pedigree with autosomal dominant type of inheritance of pathology, generation skipping is observed, i.e. a situation when phenotypically generations "slip through", i.e. individuals with an affected ancestor have affected descendants as well.

However, it should be noted that a detailed study of the phenotype can identify symptoms of hereditary disease that are not of important clinical significance, but are manifestations of a specific abnormal gene. For example, dimples on the mucosa of the lower lip in Van der Wood syndrome. On the other hand, the improvement of laboratory and instrumental methods of research makes it possible to detect other manifestations of gene functioning at clinical, biochemical and molecular levels in healthy carriers.

In general, based on modern ideas about the functioning of genes, it can be argued that if a mutant gene is present in the human genotype, its phenotypic effects can be detected. All this speaks about the conventionality of the concept of penetrance. Nevertheless, when analysing a family situation, the phenomenon of penetrance can be a very useful tool to conclude about the hereditary nature of pathology in the family.

The concept of ***expressiveness*** refers to the symptoms of the disease and reflects the degree of their expression. For example, in one of the autosomal dominant syndromes, Holt-Oram syndrome (hand-heart syndrome), the characteristic bone lesion may vary from a slightly underdeveloped radius to its absence with the formation of radial club hand.

An example of the varying expressiveness of the disease is also the differences in the severity of the course of such a frequent autosomal dominant inherited disease as neurofibromatosis. Very often, even in the same family, there are patients with a mild course (presence of pigment spots, a small number of neurofibromas, "freckles" in the skin folds) and a severe course of the disease (with CNS tumours, neurofibromas ossification and other "threatening" symptoms).

3.4. CHROMOSOMAL THEORY OF HEREDITY

In 1902-1903, the American cytologist W. Setton and the German cytologist T. Boveri independently noted parallelism in the behaviour of genes and chromosomes during gamete formation and fertilisation. These observations provided the basis for the assumption of the location of genes in chromosomes. However, experimental proof of the localisation of specific genes in specific chromosomes was obtained only in 1910 by the American geneticist T. Morgan, who in the following years (1911-1926) substantiated the *chromosomal theory of heredity*. According to this theory, the transmission of hereditary information is connected with chromosomes, in which genes are localised linearly in a certain sequence. Thus, chromosomes are the material basis of heredity.

Linked inheritance and the phenomenon of crossing over. Independent combination of traits (G. Mendel's third law) takes place provided that the genes determining these traits are located in different pairs of homologous chromosomes. Consequently, in each organism, the number of genes that can combine independently in meiosis is limited by the number of chromosome pairs. However, in an organism, the number of genes is

usually much greater than the number of chromosomes.
For example, more than 500 genes have been studied in maize, more than 1000 in the fly Drosophila, and several thousand genes in humans, while the number of chromosomes in them is 10, 4 and 23 pairs, respectively. This suggests that there are many genes localised in each chromosome. *Genes localised in one chromosome form a linkage group and are inherited together.*
T. Morgan proposed to call the joint inheritance of genes *as linked inheritance.* The number of linkage groups corresponds to the haploid set of chromosomes. A human has 23 pairs of chromosomes and 23 linkage groups, a pea has 7 pairs of chromosomes and 7 linkage groups, etc. The mode of inheritance of linked genes differs from the inheritance of genes localised in different pairs of homologous chromosomes.

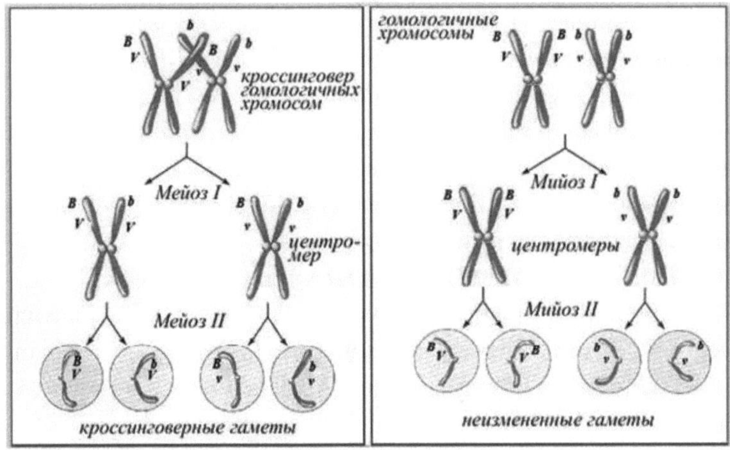

Figure 27. Complete linkage of genes. **Fig. 28.** Incomplete linkage of genes.
Thus, if at independent combination dihybrid BbVv forms four types of gametes BV, Bv, bV, bv in equal amounts, then the same dihybrid BbVv forms only two types of gametes: BV and bv also in equal amounts, which repeat the combination of genes in the chromosome of the parent.
The reason for this result is that the genes that cause the two traits are localised in the same chromosome. This phenomenon is called ***complete gene fusion*** (Figure 27). It was found that, in addition to normal gametes, other Bv and bV - with new combinations of genes, different from the parent gamete - also arise.
The cause of new gametes is the exchange of sections of homologous chromosomes, or crossingover. It's labelled:

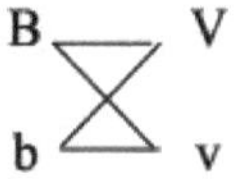

B V

b v

Crossingover occurs in prophase I of meiosis during conjugation of homologous chromosomes. At this time, parts of two chromosomes can cross and exchange their sections. As a result, qualitatively new chromosomes containing sections (genes) of both maternal and paternal chromosomes arise. The individuals that are obtained from such gametes with a new combination of alleles are called *crossing-over* or *recombinant.* This phenomenon is called *incomplete gene linkage* (Figure 28). The frequency (percentage) of crossing over between two genes located on the same chromosome is proportional to the distance between them. Crossingover between two genes occurs less frequently the closer together they are located. As the distance between genes increases, it becomes increasingly likely that crossingover will breed them on two different homologous chromosomes. The distance between genes characterises the *strength of the linkage* and is expressed in *morganids* (after T. Morgan) or percentage of recombination. The genetic distance at which crossingover occurs with a probability of 1% is *centimorgan (cM).*

Let us consider three genes A, B and C, which are inherited cross-linked, i.e. they are in the same linkage group. In a dihybrid cross, the frequencies of crossingover between them are as follows: A-B-5%, A-C-12%, B-C-7%. What is the probable order of the genes?

He could be like this:

5% 7%

A - B — C

12%

Numerous data obtained on well-studied genetic objects confirm the validity of the above example, with only one reservation. The distance A - C is equal to the sum of distances A - B, B - C in the case of closely located genes. As the distance increases, deviations are observed. Consequently, the linked genes are arranged in a linear order in the chromosome and the frequency of crossover between them is directly proportional to the distance.

Thus, the distance between genes in a chromosome is judged by the frequency of crossing over. There are genes with a high percentage of linkage and those where linkage is almost undetectable.

However, in coupled inheritance, the maximum value of crossingover does not exceed 50%. If it is higher, then free combination between pairs of alleles is observed, indistinguishable from independent inheritance. The biological significance of crossing-over is extremely high, since genetic recombination makes it possible to create new, previously non-existent combinations of genes and thereby ensure increased survival of organisms in the process of evolution.

3.4.1. HUMAN CHROMOSOME MAPS

The linkage of genes localised in one chromosome is not absolute. Crossingover, which occurs during meiosis between homologous chromosomes, leads to recombination of genes. T. Morgan and his collaborators K. Bridges, A. Sturtevang and G. Miller experimentally showed that knowledge of the phenomena of linkage and crossingover allows not only to establish the groups of gene linkage, but also to construct genetic maps of chromosomes, which indicate the order of genes in the chromosome and the relative distances between them.

A genetic map of chromosomes is a diagram of the mutual arrangement of genes that are in the same linkage group. Genetic maps are made for each pair of homologous chromosomes.

The possibility of such mapping is based on the constancy of the percentage of crossingover between certain genes. If the mutual arrangement of genes on a chromosome (their order and distance between them) is known, it can be depicted in the form of a diagram (see Appendix 1).

Classical methods for studying linkage groups developed in Drosophila are not applicable to humans because of the impossibility of direct crosses.

Therefore, only three autosomal and X chromosomal linkage groups were known in humans until the end of the 1960s. Then new methods of studying linkage, such as genetic analyses of somatic hybrid cells, became available to geneticists.

The study of morphological variants and anomalies of chromosomes, hybridisation of nucleic acids on cytological preparations, analysis of amino acid sequence of proteins and others, which allowed to describe all 23 linkage groups in humans.

One of the main goals of human genome research is to construct an accurate and detailed map of each chromosome. A genetic map shows the relative location of genes and other genetic markers on a chromosome, as well as the relative distance between them.

A genetic marker for mapping could potentially be any inherited trait, such as eye colour or DNA fragment length. The main thing in this case is the presence of easily identifiable between individual differences of the markers under consideration. Chromosome maps, like geographic maps, can be constructed at different scales and with different levels of resolution. The smallest scale map is a picture of differential chromosome staining. The maximum possible level of resolution is one nucleotide.
Hence, the largest scale map of any chromosome is the complete nucleotide sequence. The size of the human genome is approximately 3000 cM.
To date, small-scale genetic maps have been constructed for all human chromosomes with a distance between neighbouring markers of 7-10 million base pairs or 7-10 Mb (megabases; 1 Mb = 1 million base pairs). Current information on human genetic maps contains information on more than 50,000 markers.
This means that they are on average tens of thousands of base pairs away from each other, with several genes located between them. For many sites, of course, more detailed maps are available, but still most of the genes have not yet been identified and localised.
Human genetic maps can be useful in the development of health care and medicine. Knowledge about the localisation of a gene on a particular chromosome is already being used to diagnose a number of severe hereditary human diseases. Gene therapy, i.e. correction of the structure or function of genes, is already possible.

3.4.2. THEORY OF SEX INHERITANCE

In many animal species, the most prominent phenotypic difference between individuals is ***sex***. Moreover, sex affects the development and functioning of many organs not directly related to sexual reproduction, and sex hormones influence the expression of many genes.
Sex, like any other trait of an organism, is hereditarily determined. The most important role in the genetic determination of sex and in the maintenance of a regular sex ratio belongs to the chromosomal apparatus. Very long ago it was noticed that in separate-sex organisms the sex ratio is usually 1:1, i.e. males and females occur equally often. When the chromosomes of males and females, of a number of animals were studied, some differences were found between them. Both males and females have pairs of identical chromosomes in all cells, but they differ in one pair of chromosomes. Thus, the female Drosophila has two rod-shaped

chromosomes (XX), while the male has one such rod-shaped chromosome, and the second, paired with the first, is curved (XU). The chromosomes that distinguish females from males are called *sex chromosomes*, and all other chromosomes are called *autosomes*.

The female sex of most organisms forms identical gametes containing only the X chromosome and is called *homogametic.* The male sex by this feature forms gametes of two types (X and Y) and is called *heterogametic.* In some organisms (birds, butterflies, reptiles) the opposite picture is observed: female sex is heterogametic and male sex is homogametic. Sex determination in this case is usually called XU-type. In straight-winged insects, there is no U chromosome at all, so the male has the CW genotype. What does the birth of male and female individuals depend on. Let us consider this on the example of sex determination in Drosophila. During meiosis in females, one type of gametes is formed, containing a haploid set of autosomes and one X chromosome.

Males form two types of gametes, half of which contain three autosomes and one X chromosome (ZA+X) and half of which contain three autosomes and one U chromosome (ZA+U). Fertilisation of eggs (ZA+X) by spermatozoa with X chromosomes will produce females (6A+XXX), and fusion of eggs with spermatozoa carrying a U chromosome will produce males (6A+XU).

Since the number of male gametes with X and U chromosomes is the same, the number of males and females is also the same. A similar way of sex determination is inherent in all mammals, including humans.

Inheritance of sex-linked traits. The X and U chromosomes share homologous regions. These regions contain genes that determine traits that are inherited equally in both males and females (similar to autosome-linked traits).

In addition to homologous regions, the X and U chromosomes have non-homologous regions. The non-homologous region of the U chromosome contains genes for toe webbing and hairy ears, in addition to genes that determine male sex. Pathological traits linked to the non-homologous section of the U chromosome are passed on to all sons because they receive the U chromosome from their father. The non-homologous region of the X chromosome contains a number of recessive (for females) and dominant (for males - due to its hemizygosity) genes.

Examples of this type of inheritance in humans include haemophilia, optic atrophy, non-sugar diabetes, colour blindness, and baldness (Figure 29).

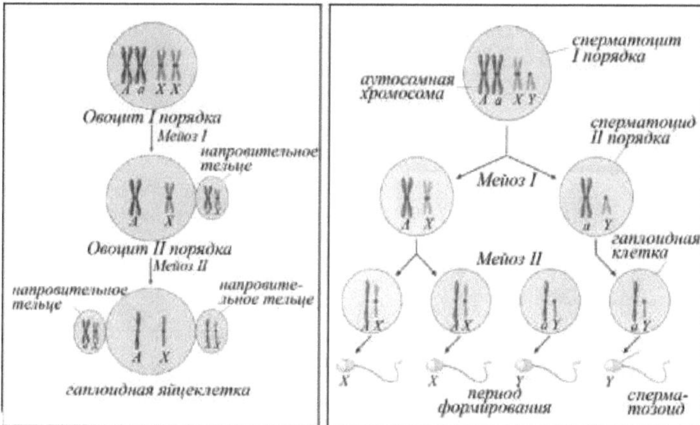

Figure 29. Schematic of sex-linked cleavage in humans (gametogenesis with autosomal and sex chromosomes).

Haemophilia is a hereditary disease in which the blood loses its ability to clot. An injury, even a scratch or bruise, can cause profuse external or internal bleeding, often resulting in death. The disease occurs, with very few exceptions, only in males. Haemophilia has been found to be caused by a recessive gene localised in the X chromosome, so women heterozygous for this gene have normal blood clotting.

Let us consider what kind of offspring can be born to a woman who marries a man who is normal in this respect. The gene that determines normal blood coagulation is labelled H, and the gene that determines its incompatibility is labelled h. Taking into account that in the genotype of a woman there are two X chromosomes, and in men - one X chromosome and one U chromosome, let us write down the scheme of haemophilia inheritance:

P: X^HX^h x X^Hy

haemophilia gene carrier healthy

Gametes X^H, X^h X^H, y

F$_1$: $X^H X^H$; X^HX^h; X^Hy; X^hy.

healthy carrier girl carrier girl healthy carrier boy haemophiliac boy.

As can be seen from the scheme, the offspring of this marriage show a split trait: half of the daughters (X X^{Hh}) are carriers of the haemophilia gene and half of the sons are haemophiliacs; the other half - daughters (X^H X^H) and sons (X^H U) will turn out to be healthy.

The phenotypic manifestation of haemophilia in girls is observed if the girl's mother is a carrier of the haemophilia gene and the father is a haemophiliac:

P: X^HX^h x X^Hy

male host

haemophilia gene haemophiliac

Gametes: X^H, X^h X^h, y

F_1: $X^H X^h$; X^hX^h; X^Hy; X^hy.

haemophilia gene carrier girl haemophiliac girl.

a healthy haemophiliac boy

The gene causing ***colour blindness*** is also recessive, linked to the X chromosome. As for the baldness gene, it is localised in the autosome, but its expression depends on male sex hormones.

In men, this gene is dominant due to the presence of male sex hormones; in women, it behaves as a recessive gene and does not cause baldness.

Control Questions and Assignments:

1. What are genotype and phenotype? What is their relationship?
2. What is expressivity and penetrance.
3. What is the pleiotropic action of a gene?
4. What were the basic laws established by H. Mendel?
5. What are allelic genes, and what are the main types of gene interactions?
6. What are the main types of non-allelic gene interactions?
7. What is the essence of the chromosomal theory of heredity?
8. What is coupled inheritance and what are its characteristics.
9. What are the basic tenets of the chromosomal theory of heredity?

TEST-3.

1. Explain why the haemophilia gene always appears in males but is rarely seen in females?

(a)_the gene is recessive and located on the U chromosome;

b) the gene is dominant and located in the X chromosome;

(c) The gene is recessive and located on the X chromosome;

e) the gene is dominant and located in the autosome.

2. Which sex is called homogametic (a), which sex is called heterogametic (b).

1 - with two X chromosomes;

2 - with an X and a U chromosome;

3 - in humans, it's male;

4 - In the chicken, it is male.

(a)a-1,4 6-2,3; (c)a-2,3 6-1,4;
b)a-1,3 6-2,4; e)a- 2,4 6-1,3.

3. From which parent do girls inherit the condition colour blindness?
a) From the father; b) From the mother;
c) From the father and from the mother; e) Cannot be determined.

4. A woman is healthy, a man is sick. All the children in this family are healthy, but when their daughters marry a healthy man, a sick boy is born in their family. identify the type of inheritance of the trait?
a) recessive, linked to the U chromosome;
б) recessive, X-linked;
(c) Autosomal recessive type;
e) autosomal dominant type;

5. Which diseases are inherited by sex-linked inheritance
a) Klinefelter's, Down's; b) Albinism, Phenylketonuria;
c) Haemophilia, Daltonism; e) Haemophilia, Down's.

CHALLENGE-3.

1. In humans, the gene that causes a form of hereditary deafblindness is recessive to the gene for normal hearing.
a) What offspring can be expected from the marriage of heterozygous parents?
б) A deaf-mute child was born from the marriage of a deaf-mute woman with a normal man. Determine the genotypes of the parents.

2. How many types of gametes and which ones form organisms with the following genotypes:
a)aabb; b)AaBB; c)AaBb; d)AaBCC; e)AaBCC; f)AaBCC?

3. In humans, clubfoot dominates over normal foot structure and normal carbohydrate metabolism over diabetes mellitus. A woman with a normal foot structure and normal carbohydrate metabolism married a clubfooted man who also had normal carbohydrate metabolism. Two children were born from this marriage, one with only clubfoot and the other with only diabetes mellitus. Determine the probability of having a child with both abnormalities in this family.

4. Familial hypercholesterolaemia is inherited dominantly through autosomes. Heterozygotes have high blood cholesterol, while homozygotes also develop xanthomas (benign tumours) of the skin and tendons and atherosclerosis. Determine the possible degree of hypercholesterolaemia in children in a family where both parents have only high blood cholesterol.

5. A woman heterozygous for blood type A (II) married a man with blood type AB (IV). What blood types will their children have?

CHAPTER IV

HEREDITY AND ENVIRONMENT.

4.1. VARIABILITY, ITS FORMS

Earlier we defined variability as one of the most important universal properties of life, which leads to the diversity of representatives of any species. Due to this, the requirements of organisms to the living environment are somewhat different, which allows the species to disperse over large areas. Diversity also forms the basis for evolutionary changes in a species, it determines the possibility of adaptation to newly emerging conditions of existence.

Changes that appear in the phenotype of an organism and distinguish it from other members of the species may be either the result of a direct response of the organism to the influence of some environmental factors or the result of earlier changes in the hereditary material, which then manifest themselves phenotypically. Depending on this, two main forms of variability are distinguished (Fig. 30).

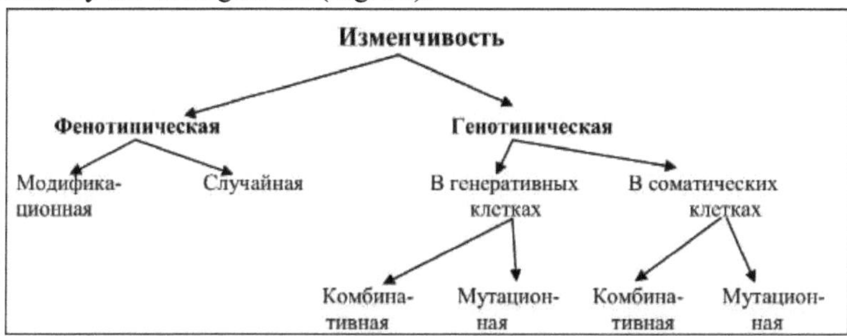

Figure 30. Classification of types of variability.

In the first case, when changes in a trait arise without prior changes in the hereditary material and represent a direct response of the organism to environmental influences, we speak *of non-heritable, modification*, or *phenotypic variability.* If phenotypic changes are a reflection of changes that have arisen initially in the hereditary material, this is *hereditary,* or *genotypic, variability.*

Variability is of great importance in the evolutionary process because it is the most important condition for the historical development of species.

4.1.1. NON-HERITABLE VARIABILITY

All the diversity of living things and its constant perfection would be impossible without variability. This is due to the fact that genotype is consistently realised into phenotype in the course of individual development and under certain environmental conditions. Various environmental factors (light, heat, moisture, soil composition, etc.) have a direct or indirect effect on organisms, causing them to change their traits and properties. This is what determines the fact that organisms with the same genotypes can differ sharply from each other in phenotype. Thus, an organism possesses not only heredity, which supplies material for evolution and selection, but also variability.

Modification (non-heritable or phenotypic) variability is an evolutionarily fixed adaptive reaction of an organism to changes in environmental conditions without changing the genotype. Modifications are not inherited and persist only during the life of a given organism.

All traits and properties of an organism are hereditarily determined, but *organisms do not inherit the traits and properties themselves, but only the possibility of their development.*

The formation of a trait, a chain of processes running from genes through iRNA, polypeptide and enzyme, proceeds normally only if the cell has all the necessary starting substances, energy source and suitable conditions for the reaction.

Thus, the environment must provide the conditions necessary for the formation of the trait.

If seeds of plants, such as cereals, or potato tubers are germinated in the light, the seedlings formed are green in colour because of the presence of chloroplasts in their cells. The same seedlings, but grown in the dark, become colourless or slightly yellowish. If they are brought back into the light, they become green in colour. Thus, the possibility of formation of chlorophyll and consequently chloroplasts was present in both cases, but light was necessary for its realisation.

But even in the case when the emergence and development of this or that trait occurs, the degree of its expression may be different depending on the environmental conditions: under some conditions it may be strengthened, under others - weakened. The limits of these changes are determined by the possibilities inherent in the genotype.

The limits of variation of a trait, limited by the action of genotype genes, are called the response norm.

In phenotypic variability, hereditary material is not involved in the changes. They concern only the manifested traits of an individual and occur under the influence of factors of the external or internal environment of the organism. Such changes are not inherited by the next generations, even if they are caused by prolonged and/or repeated influences over a historically long period of time. For example, in some peoples, initiation rites are associated with specific injuries: piercing of the nasal septum and lips, removal of fangs, circumcision of the foreskin, disfigurement of the feet or skull bones, etc. Such changes are not known to be inherited. They are only a reaction to the action of a certain factor. If the expression of changes in the organism does not go beyond the normal reaction, such changes in the phenotype are called *modification* changes. Modification variability has adaptive (adaptive) significance. Modification variability is most clearly revealed when studying the reactions of the organism to changes in environmental factors: for example, living conditions in different geographical zones, the intensity of solar radiation, the nature of nutrition, etc. Previously, it was believed that changes in phenotype that are not associated with genetic changes have no evolutionary significance. However, this view is not correct, because the degree and direction of acceptable phenotypic variability is strictly controlled by the genetic constitution of the organism.

Thus, genes determine the possibility of trait development in individuals within certain limits. The final result in the form of a certain degree of expression of a trait depends on the conditions in which the organism develops. Different traits are capable of modification under the influence of environmental conditions to different degrees. For example, the formation of the trait of blood group belonging to the ABO system practically does not depend on environmental conditions, but is entirely determined by a specific combination of genes in the human organism.

One of the manifestations of modification variability is the phenomenon of phenocopying. The term *phenocopying* was proposed to denote traits, diseases or malformations that develop under the influence of certain environmental conditions but are phenotypically similar to the same conditions caused by genetic factors (mutations).

Thus, phenocopy is a trait developing under the influence of environmental factors, but only copying a heritable trait.

Thus, the skin colouration of Africans is characterised by pronounced pigmentation, even if the person is not exposed to sunlight. The skin of Europeans, as a rule, is pigmented only to a weak degree, but becomes swarthy under the influence of light. Thus, tanned but hereditarily fair-skinned individuals are like "copies" of genetically dark-skinned people. There are many clinical examples illustrating situations where a particular phenotype may be a product of a particular genotype, or it may be a phenocopy, i.e. developed under the influence of environmental factors. For example, blindness due to clouding of the lens of the eye (cataract) may be caused by mechanical damage or the action of ionising radiation, or as a result of intrauterine infection with rubella virus. But the development of cataracts can be caused by a specific gene, without any additional external influence on the organism.

Dementia may be due to a specific genotype (e.g., a gene or genomic mutation), but can develop when iodine is not present in a child's diet or as a result of the damaging effects of cytomegalovirus infection on the fetal brain during intrauterine development.

In some cases, the term used reflects only the presence of a feature and does not carry information about the causes of its occurrence. It is known, for example, that the term "microcephaly" (from Greek *mikros* - small + *kephale* - head) includes such features as reduced size of the skull and brain, mental retardation and certain neurological disorders. But microcephaly can be *true,* or *genetic*, characterised by primary underdevelopment of the brain, and *secondary,* or non-genetic, *caused,* for example, by early accretion of cranial sutures. In both cases, many of the clinical manifestations will be quite similar. However, when choosing methods of psychological and pedagogical correction, therapy, rehabilitation and adaptation of these patients, it is necessary to know the exact cause of pathology in a given family. Formed new traits can serve as a basis for the evolution of the species, provided that they are inherited.

If all members of a species were identical in some way, there would be no selection because there would be no point of application of its 91
action. The phenomenon of variability thus enables natural selection. However, evolution requires not just variability, but inherited variability in order to be able to propagate the changes that are beneficial or remove those that are harmful to the species. The most important thing for evolutionary transformations of the genetic structure of a species is that individuals differing in genetic constitution leave different numbers of descendants. This determines the basic mechanism of evolution.

Because modification changes are adaptive in nature, they provide a greater probability of survival for organisms with a broad norm of genotype response under changing conditions of existence.

4.1.2. HEREDITARY VARIABILITY

Hereditary variability is caused by changes in genetic material and is the basis of the diversity of living organisms, as well as the main cause of the evolutionary process, as it supplies material for natural selection.

Genotypic variability, depending on the nature of cells, is divided into *generative* (changes in the hereditary apparatus of gametes) and *somatic* (changes in the hereditary apparatus of body cells). Within generative and somatic variability, 1) combinative and 2) mutational variability are distinguished.

The basis of *combinatorial variability* is the sexual process, which results in a huge set of diverse genotypes. The cells of each individual contain 23 maternal and 23 paternal chromosomes. When forming gametes, only 23 chromosomes will fall into each of them, and how many of them will be from the father and how many from the mother is a matter of chance. This is the first source of combinatorial variability.

Its second cause is crossingover. Not only does each of our cells carry the chromosomes of our grandparents, but a certain part of these chromosomes has received, as a result of crossingover, part of its genes from homologous chromosomes that previously belonged to another line of ancestors. Such chromosomes are called *recombinative* chromosomes. Participating in the formation of the organism of a new generation, they lead to unexpected combinations of traits that were not present in either the paternal or maternal organism.

Finally, the third cause of combinatorial variability is the random nature of the encounters of certain gametes during fertilisation. All three processes underlying combinatorial variability act independently of each other, creating a huge variety of all kinds of genotypes. The occurrence of changes in the hereditary material, i.e. in DNA molecules, is called *mutational variability*. Moreover, changes can occur both in individual molecules (chromosomes) and in the number of these molecules. Mutation occurs under the influence of various factors of external and internal environment.

The term *"mutation"* was first proposed in 1901 by the Dutch scientist G. De Fries, who described spontaneous mutations in plants. Mutations appear rarely, but lead to sudden abrupt changes in traits that are transmitted from generation to generation.

The main points of the mutation theory are summarised as follows:

- mutations occur suddenly as discrete changes in traits;
- the new forms are sustainable;
- unlike non-heritable changes, mutations do not form a continuous

series. They represent qualitative changes;

- mutations manifest themselves in different ways and can be both beneficial and harmful;
- the probability of detecting mutations depends on the number of individuals studied;
- similar mutations can occur repeatedly;
- mutations are non-directional (spontaneous), i.e. any part of the chromosome can mutate, causing changes in both minor and vital traits (Fig. 31).

The factor that induced the mutation is called a mutagen.

According to their nature, 3 groups of mutagens are distinguished:

1. Physical factors (ionising radiation, gamma rays, X-rays). At the beginning of our century it was shown that *ionising radiation has* a strong mutagenic effect. A dose of 10P doubles the frequency of mutations in humans. That is why the problem of nuclear energy development attracts close attention of specialists - biologists and medics.

The evolution of life on Earth for several billion years took place in the conditions of natural background radiation created by cosmic radiation, u-radiation of the Earth, gaseous radioactive element radon. Nowadays, as a result of human industrial activity in some territories of the Earth the radiation background is 2 times higher than the norm. Nuclear explosions and industrial radioactive sources pollute the environment with strontium (^{90} Sr) and other radioactive elements, which accumulate in soil, plants, get into water. In any case, nuclear explosions are an additional source of radiation, which is a factor that can significantly affect the health of present and future generations.

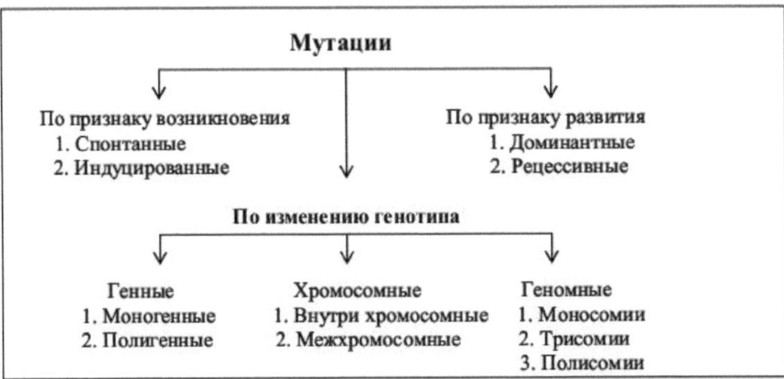

Mutations

By origin

1. Spontaneous
2. Induced
By development
1. Dominant
2. Recessive
By genotype change

Genes
1. Monogenic
2. Polygenic
Chromosomal
1. Intrachromosomal
2. Interchromosomal
Genomic
1. Monosomies
2. Trisomies
3. Polysemy

Figure 31. Schematic of mutation types.

2 **Chemical compounds** used in agriculture: herbicides and pesticides (DDT), in medicine as drugs (thiazine derivatives, formalin, etc.), in various industries (afoxide-impregnator of textile fabrics, sodium bisulphite - preservative of wines in the food industry).

Rapid development of science and technology has caused the appearance of a large number of *chemical compounds,* many of which are capable of affecting heredity material and are characterised by high mutagenic activity. These compounds directly or indirectly get into the organism of animals and humans through air, water, food, medicines, food additives, preservatives, etc. Some chemical compounds pose a greater mutagenic hazard than radiation.

Such compounds include many pesticides (hexachlorobenzene, etc.), nitrates, the source of which are mainly mineral fertilisers. At present, the widespread use of pesticides and fertilisers poses a difficult task for researchers: to find ways to protect food and humans from these mutagens entering the environment. Some food additives and preservatives, such as formalin, propylene glycol, vanillin, potassium nitrate, sodium nitrate have mutagenic properties.

In this regard, the modern canning industry represents a significant source of mutagens for humans. The mutagenicity of caffeine contained in tea and coffee, as well as in some soft drinks and medicines, has been proven.

3. biological objects (viruses, protozoa, helminths). When penetrating into the human body can cause disruption of the DNA structure of cells.

In addition to physical and chemical, there are biological factors of mutagenesis. These include viruses such as: AIDS, measles, influenza and rubella, which affect the system that shields DNA from damage, altering the frequency of mutations in the host. Viruses create a constant flow of foreign DNA into animal, plant and human cells, causing mutations in them. Some live vaccines with suppressed virulence have mutagenic properties, as well as various toxins of biological nature formed by parasites - protozoa and helminths, which are able to modify mutagenesis in the host organism. Events leading to the emergence of mutations are called the mutational process.

4.1.3. TYPES OF MUTATIONS

Mutations can be grouped into groups classified by the nature of manifestation, by place or level of their occurrence. In principle, there is no difference between the mutations assigned to one or another group, as they are combined based on convenience.

Mutations are the initial link in the pathogenesis of hereditary diseases. According to the type of cells in which the changes occurred, mutations can be divided into:

Generative - mutations in germ cells. They are inherited and, as a rule, are found in all cells of the offspring who became their carriers;

Somatic - mutations in the non-sex cells of the organism. They are manifested in the individual in which they occur. They are transmitted only to daughter cells during division and are not inherited by the next generation of the individual. If a somatic mutation occurs early in zygote division (but not the first division), cell lines with different genotypes arise. The earlier in ontogenesis a somatic mutation occurs, the more cells and consequently tissues carry the mutation. Such organisms are called mosaic organisms.

The distinction is made on the basis of origin: *spontaneous* and *induced* mutagenesis. The division of the mutational process into spontaneous and induced to a certain extent is conditional.

Spontaneous mutations - arise under normal physiological conditions of the organism without visible additional impact of external factors on the organism. Spontaneous mutations can arise, for example, as a result of the action of chemical compounds formed in the process of metabolism, the effects of natural background radiation or UV radiation, replication errors, etc.

Induced mutations are mutations caused by the directed influence of external or internal environmental factors. Induced mutation process can be controlled (e.g., in an experiment to study the action of mechanisms or its consequences) and uncontrolled (e.g., as a result of irradiation when radioactive elements are released into the environment).

Developmental traits: can be *dominant* or *recessive.* Most of them are recessive and do not appear in heterozygotes. This is very important for the existence of the species. Mutations are, as a rule, harmful, as they introduce disturbances in a finely balanced system of biochemical transformations. Possessors of harmful dominant mutations, immediately manifested in homo- and heterozygous organism, often appear unviable and die at the earliest stages of ontogenesis. If they survive, they have reduced viability or fecundity (do not leave offspring). We can give an example of the disease *achondroplasia or chondrodystrophy.* Diseases of the bone system.

Achondroplasia is an inherited disorder associated with very short stature (Fig. 32). A large head with a protruding forehead and midface hypoplasia, in which the midface is underdeveloped, is typical. It is usually characterised by short arms and legs, while the trunk is only slightly smaller than normal.

This disease has been known about for several thousand years, but was first used in 1878 by French physician M.J.Parro (M.J.Parro).

However, strictly speaking, this term is not accurate because cartilage formation in achondroplasia is generally normal and the growth disorder is caused by abnormalities in the growth zones of the skeleton. This mutation causes a change in the growth factor receptor, causing a signal to slow bone growth. The receptor is thought to be found in all growth zones of the skeleton. The reason why it affects the arm and leg areas in particular is unknown. Achondroplasia is characterised by an autosomal dominant type of inheritance. This means that if at least one parent has a genetically determined disease, there is a 50 per cent chance that the disease will be passed on to the child. Boys and girls get the disease at the same rate. Children who have not passed on the mutated gene do not have the disease and do not pass it on.

The vast majority of inherited disorders are caused by a new mutation. This means that the genetic mutation occurs for the first time in a person, rather than being passed on from one of the parents. Hence, for parents who have a child

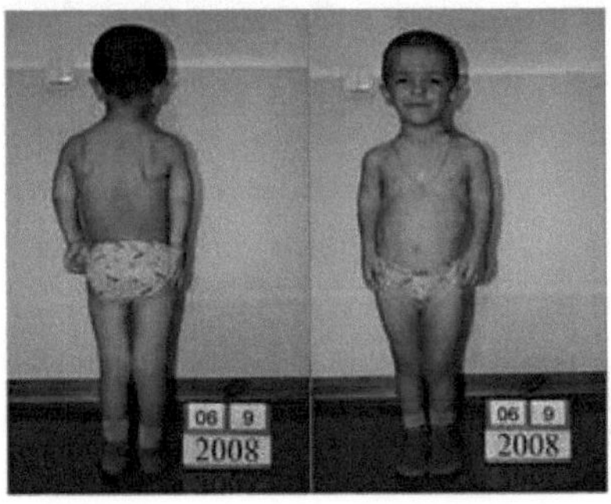

With a new mutation, there is usually no increased risk that another child will have the disease. However, new genetic mutations will be inherited, and an adult woman or adult man with the mutation is at risk of passing the mutated gene to her children.

Figure 32: Achondroplasia or chondrodystrophy.

The type of inheritance in this case is already autosomnodominant. According to the effect on the organism, it can be distinguished:

1) Lethal mutations are mutations that cause intrauterine death or death in infancy. For example, a genomic mutation such as autosomal monosomy in humans is incompatible with normal embryonic development;

2) Semi-lethal mutations are mutations that significantly reduce the viability of the organism, leading to early death. Life expectancy of carriers of semi-legal mutations can vary significantly, but in any case they die before reaching puberty (for example, in pigmentary xeroderma); ***Neutral mutations*** - mutations that do not significantly affect the processes of vital activity;

3) Favourable mutations are mutations that provide the organism with new beneficial properties.

According to the level of organisation of hereditary structures*, gene, chromosomal and genomic* mutations are distinguished.

Gene or **point mutations are the** result of a change in the nucleotide sequence of a DNA molecule in a particular region of the chromosome. Such a change in the sequence of nitrogenous bases in a given gene is reproduced during transcription in the structure of iRNA and leads to a change in the sequence of amino acids in the polypeptide chain formed as a result of translation on ribosomes. There are different types of gene mutations associated with the addition, deletion or rearrangement of nucleotides in a gene. These are duplications, insertions of an extra pair of nucleotides, deletions (loss of a pair of nucleotides), inversions or substitutions of nucleotide pairs

(AT^GC; AT^CG or AT^TA).

The effects of gene mutations are extremely diverse. Most small gene mutations are not phenotypically manifested (because they are recessive), but there are a number of cases in which a change of just one base in a particular gene has a profound effect on phenotype. One example is sickle cell anaemia, a disease caused in humans by a base substitution in one of the genes responsible for haemoglobin synthesis. This causes red blood cells with such haemoglobin to become deformed (from rounded to sickle-shaped) and rapidly deteriorate in the blood. This causes acute anaemia and reduces the amount of oxygen carried by the blood. Anaemia causes physical weakness and can even lead to heart and kidney disorders and early death in people homozygous for the mutant allele.

Gene mutations occur under the influence of ultraviolet rays, ionising radiation, chemical mutagens and other factors. Especially the ionising radiation background of our planet has a negative effect. Even a small increase in the natural background radiation (by 1/3), for example, as a result of nuclear weapons tests, can lead to the emergence in each generation an additional 20 million people with severe hereditary disorders. It is not difficult to imagine what danger not only for the population of Ukraine, Belarus and Russia, but also for mankind such events as the accident at Chernobyl NPP represent.

It is gene mutations that cause the development of most hereditary forms of pathology. Diseases caused by such mutations are called gene or monogenic diseases, i.e. diseases whose development is determined by a single gene mutation. Monogenic diseases include: cystic fibrosis, phenylketonuria, haemophilia, neurofibromatosis, Duchenne-Becker myopathy and many other diseases.

Chromosomal mutations, or **chromosomal rearrangements**, are expressed as changes in the structure of chromosomes that can be detected and studied under a light microscope. A large number (tens to several hundred) of genes are involved in a chromosomal mutation, resulting in a change in the normal diploid set. Although chromosomal aberrations usually do not alter the DNA sequence in specific genes, the change in the number of gene copies in the genome leads to genetic imbalance due to a deficiency or excess of genetic material. Two large groups of chromosomal mutations are distinguished: intra-chromosomal and interchromosomal.

Intrachromosomal mutations are aberrations within a single chromosome. They include:

- *deficiencies,* or *deficienciesci,* is the loss of the end portions of a chromosome;
- *deletions* - loss of a section of a chromosome in the middle part of the chromosome;

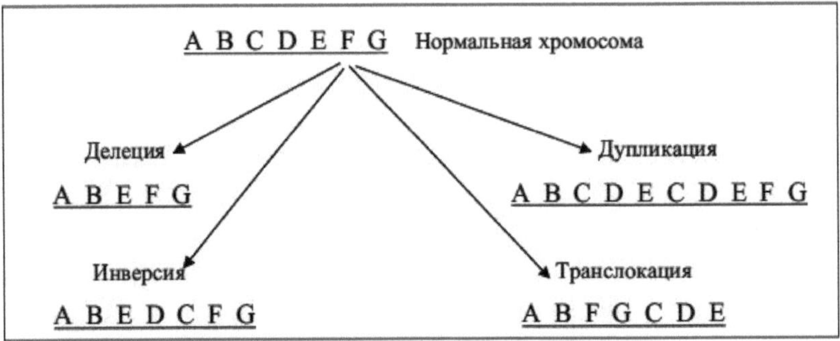

Fig. 33 Schematic of a chromosomal mutation

- *duplications* - two or multiple repetitions of a set of genes localised in a particular region of the chromosome;
- *inversions* - turning a section of a chromosome by 18O ;^{0}
- *translocation* - transfer of a site to the other end of the same chromosome or to another non-homologous chromosome (Figure 33).

Deficiencies, deletions and duplications change the amount of genetic material in the chromosomes. The extent of the phenotypic change depends on how large the relevant chromosome regions are and whether they contain important genes. Examples of chromosomal rearrangements are known in many organisms, including humans.

A *deletion* (from Latin *deletio* - destruction) or loss of one of the chromosome regions, internal or terminal. This can cause disruption of embryogenesis and the formation of multiple developmental anomalies (for example, a deletion in the region of the short arm of the 5th chromosome, designated as 5p-, leads to underdevelopment of the larynx, heart defects, mental retardation). This severe hereditary disease "cat cry" syndrome (named so by the nature of the sounds made by sick infants) is caused by heterozygosity for a division in the 5th chromosome. This syndrome is accompanied by mental retardation. Usually children with this syndrome die early.

Duplications (from Latin *duplicatio* - doubling) - multiplication of any part of a chromosome (for example, trisomy on one of the short arms of the 9th chromosome causes multiple defects, including microcephaly, delayed physical, mental and intellectual development, play a significant role in the evolution of the genome, as they can serve as material for the emergence of new genes, as different mutational processes can occur in each of the two previously identical sites.

Interchromosomal mutations or rearrangement mutations are the exchange of fragments between non-homologous chromosomes. Such mutations are called *translocations* (from Latin *tzans* - behind, through + *locus* - place). These are:

- *reciprocal translocation*, when two chromosomes exchange their fragments;
- *Non-reciprocal translocation*, where a fragment of one chromosome is transported to another;
- *"centric"* fusion (Robertsonian translocation) - fusion of two acrocentric chromosomes near their centromeres with loss of short arms.

When chromatids are transversely separated through centromeres, the "sister" chromatids become the "mirror" arms of two different chromosomes containing the same sets of genes. Such chromosomes are called *isochromosomes.*

In inversions and translocations, the total amount of genetic material remains the same, only its location changes. Such mutations also play a significant role in evolution, since crossing mutants with the original forms is difficult, and their hybrids F_1 are most often sterile. Therefore, only crossing of the original forms among themselves is possible here. If such mutants have a favourable phenotype, they can become the initial forms for the origin of new species. In humans, all of these mutations lead to pathological conditions. Genomic and chromosomal mutations are the causes of chromosomal diseases.

Genomic mutations. These include aneuploidies and ploidy changes in structurally unchanged chromosomes. They are detected by cytogenetic methods.

Aneuploidy is a change (decrease - monosomy, increase - trisomy) in the number of chromosomes in the diploid set, not multiple of the haploid one (2n +1,2p - 1, etc.).

Polyploidy is an increase in the number of chromosome sets that is a multiple of the haploid number (Zp, 4p, 5p, etc.). In humans, polyploidy and most aneuploidies are lethal mutations. The most frequent genomic mutations include: trisomy - the presence of three homologous chromosomes in the karyotype (for example, on the 21st pair in Down syndrome, on the 18th pair in Edwards syndrome, on the 13th pair in Patau syndrome; on sex chromosomes: XXX, XXY, XYY).

Monosomy is the presence of only one of two homologous chromosomes. In case of monosomy on any of the autosomes, normal development of the embryo is impossible. The only monosomy in humans that is compatible with life is monosomy on the X chromosome, which leads to Sherechevsky-Turner syndrome (45, XO). The main mechanisms underlying aneuploidy are *chromosome divergence* during cell division in the formation of germ cells, and *loss of chromosomes* as a result of "anaphase lag" when one homologous chromosome may lag behind all other non-homologous chromosomes during movement to the pole. The term *"non-disjunction"* refers to the lack of separation of chromosomes or chromatids in meiosis or mitosis. Loss of chromosomes can lead to mosaicism, in which there is one euploid (normal) cell line and another monosomal cell line. Chromosome missegregation is most commonly observed during meiosis (Figure 34).

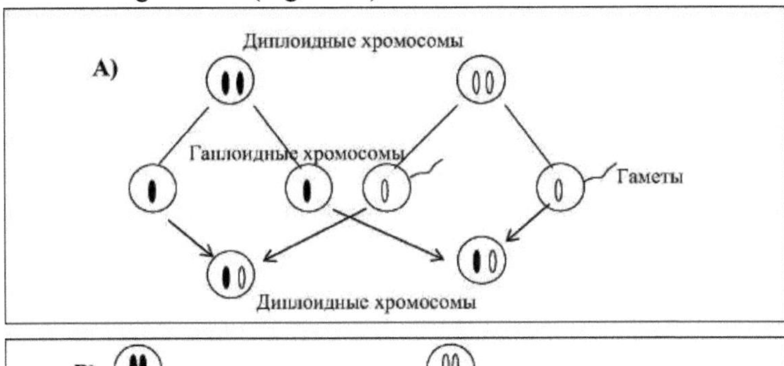

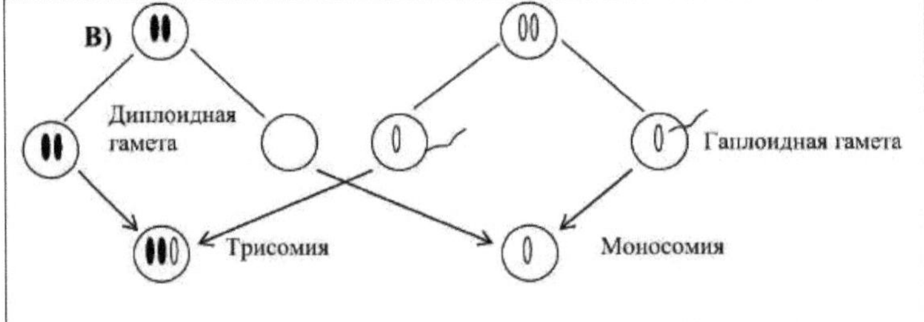

Figure 34. Cytological mechanism of genomic mutations.
A) proper distribution of gametes; B) improper distribution of gametes.

In humans, for reasons unknown so far, non-disjunction is most often found on acrocentric chromosomes. The chromosomes, which normally should divide during meiosis, remain joined together and in anaphase move to one pole of the cell. In this way, two gametes arise, one of which has an extra chromosome and the other does not have this chromosome. When a gamete with a normal set of chromosomes is fertilised by a gamete with an "extra" chromosome, trisomy occurs (i.e. there are three homologous chromosomes in the cell), and when a gamete is fertilised by a gamete without one chromosome, a zygote with monosomy occurs. If a monosomic zygote is formed by any autosomal (non-sex) chromosome, the development of the organism stops at the earliest stages of development.

4.1.4. HEREDITARY PATHOLOGY AS A RESULT OF HEREDITARY VARIABILITY

The presence of common species traits allows us to unite all people on earth into a single species Homo sapiens. Nevertheless, we can easily, with a single glance, distinguish the face of a familiar person in a crowd of strangers. The extreme diversity of people - both intra-group (e.g. diversity within an ethnos) and inter-group - is due to their genetic differences. It is currently believed that all intraspecific variability is due to different genotypes arising and maintained by natural selection.

It is known that the haploid human genome contains $3.Zx10^9$ pairs of nucleotide residues, which theoretically allows to have up to 6-10 million genes. At the same time the data of modern researches testify that the human genome contains approximately 30-40 thousand genes. About one third of all genes have more than one allele, i.e. they are polymorphic.

The concept of hereditary polymorphism was formulated by E. Ford in 1940 to explain the existence of two or more divergent forms in a population when the frequency of the rarest of them cannot be explained by mutational events alone. Since a gene mutation is a rare event ($1x10^{-6}$), the frequency of the mutant allele, which is more than 1%, can only be explained by its gradual accumulation in the population due to the selective advantages of carriers of this mutation.

The multiplicity of cleavage loci, the multiplicity of alleles in each of them, along with the phenomenon of recombination, creates an inexhaustible genetic diversity of human beings. Calculations testify that for the whole history of mankind on the globe there was not, is not and in the foreseeable future will not meet genetic repetition, i.e. each born person is a unique phenomenon in the Universe. The uniqueness of genetic constitution largely determines the peculiarities of disease development in each individual.

Humankind evolved as groups of isolated populations living for a long time in the same environmental conditions, including climatogeographical characteristics, nutritional patterns, pathogens, cultural traditions, etc. This led to the consolidation in the population of combinations of normal alleles specific to each of them, which are most adequate to the environmental conditions.

Due to the gradual expansion of the habitat, intensive migrations, and resettlement of peoples, situations arise when combinations of specific normal genes that are useful in certain conditions do not ensure optimal functioning of some organism systems in other conditions. This leads to the fact that the part of hereditary variability caused by unfavourable combinations of non-pathological human genes becomes the basis for the development of so-called diseases with hereditary predisposition.

In addition, in man as a social creature, natural selection took more and more specific forms over time, which also expanded hereditary diversity. What could be cancelled out in animals was retained, or, conversely, what animals retained was lost. For example, the full provision of vitamin C requirements led in the course of evolution to the loss of the gene for L-gulonodac-tonoxidase, which catalyses the synthesis of ascorbic acid.

In the process of evolution, mankind has also acquired undesirable traits that are directly related to pathology. For example, in the course of evolution, humans have acquired genes that determine sensitivity to diphtheria toxin or poliomyelitis virus.

There is also a mechanism of genetic variability associated with resistance to certain diseases. It is known that heterozygous carriage of sickle cell haemoglobin (HbS) provides the human body with protection against malaria plasmodium (an intracellular parasite of red blood cells). Although HbS homozygotes suffer severe anaemia and usually die at an early age, the HbS gene carrier is a beneficial trait for the general population, and the frequency of the mutant gene can reach high values in malaria-endemic settings.

Thus, in humans, as in any other biological species, there is no sharp boundary between hereditary variability leading to normal variations of traits and hereditary variability causing the emergence of hereditary diseases. Man, having become the biological species *"Homo sapiens"*, as it were, paid for the "reasonableness" of his species by the accumulation of pathological mutations. This position is the basis of one of the main concepts of medical genetics about evolutionary accumulation of pathological mutations in human populations.

Hereditary variability in human populations, both maintained and reduced by natural selection, forms the so-called genetic load. Some pathological mutations may persist and spread in populations for a historically long time, causing the so-called segregation genetic load; other pathological mutations arise in each generation as a result of new changes in hereditary structure, creating a mutation load.

The negative effects of genetic load are manifested by increased lethality (death of gametes, zygotes, embryos and children), reduced fertility (reduced reproduction of offspring), reduced life expectancy, social maladaptation and disability, and increased need for medical care.

The English geneticist J. Hoddane was the first to draw the attention of researchers to the existence of genetic load, although the term itself was proposed by G. Meller in the late 40s. The meaning of the concept of "genetic load" is associated with a high degree of genetic variability necessary for a biological species to be able to adapt to changing environmental conditions.

Control Questions and Assignments:

1. Give a definition of the term "variability"?
2. What are the main features of modification variability?
3. What is the fundamental difference between phenotypic and genotypic variability?
4. Explain the term "phenocopying".
5. Give examples of physical, chemical and biological mutagens.
6. What constitutes gene mutations?
7. Give a definition of genomic mutations?
8. Give a definition of chromosomal mutations.
9. Give examples of chromosomal mutations.
10. What are the mechanisms underlying genomic mutations?

TEST-4.

1. By whom and in what year was the theory of mutation put forward?

a) V. Johansen in 1903 b) Hugo de. Fries in 1901 - 1903.

c) G.A.Nadsonomi G.S.Phillipov in 1925 e) Meller in 1927.

2. Indicate the correspondence between the types of mutations and the examples that characterise them.

1) brochidactyly; 2) duplication; 3) haemophilia; 4) inversion
5) increase in the number of chromosomes;6) polyploidy.
a) gene mutations; b) chromosomal mutations; c) genomic mutations;
a) a-1,3 6-2,4 c-5,6; b) a-2,3 6-4,5 c-1,6;
(c) a-1,4 6-2,6 d-3,5; e) a-3,5 6-1,4 c-2,6.
3. What is a mutation in humans that is incompatible with normal embryo development called?
(a) favourable mutation6) neutral mutation
(c) Lethal mutation (d) Semi-legal mutation
4. In which syndrome are low-set auricles, narrow eye slits, and a short mandible observed?
(a) Edwards syndrome; 6) Patau syndrome;
(c) Down syndrome; (d) Catcall syndrome.
5. Identify the correct statement for a healthy woman whose dad is colour blind and whose mum is healthy.
a) 100% of sons will be healthy from marrying a sick man;
б) the sister is homozygous and healthy;
(c) 100 per cent of sons will be healthy from marriage to a healthy man;
e) 100% of daughters will be healthy from marriage to a healthy man.

CHALLENGE-4.

1. All cells of a sick man have 47 chromosomes due to an extra X chromosome. Specify the name of this mutation, all possible mechanisms of its occurrence and the probability of its transmission to offspring.
2. A man is phenotypically healthy, but he has a balanced translocation of chromosome 21 to chromosome 15. Can this mutation affect his offspring?
3. Genes affecting Rh antigen protein synthesis and red blood cell shape are located in the same autosome at a distance of 3 morganids. A woman whose father was Rh negative but had elliptical erythrocytes (dominant trait) and whose mother is Rh positive, with normal erythrocytes, has elliptical erythrocytes and is Rh positive. Her husband is Rh negative, with normal red blood cells. Determine the probability of having a baby:
a) Rhesus-positive with normal red blood cells;
б) Rhesus-positive with elliptical erythrocytes;
в) Rh-negative with elliptical erythrocytes;
г) Rh-negative with normal red blood cells.
4. A woman who contracted measles rubella during pregnancy gave birth to a deaf son. She and her husband have normal hearing, and there is no history of deafness in the pedigrees of either spouse. Determine the

possible mechanism of deafness in the child; the probability of repeated birth of a deaf child in this family; the probability of deaf grandchildren if their deaf son, as an adult, marries a deaf-mute woman whose parents and both sisters are also deaf-mute (the gene for deafness is recessive).

5. Edik was born with phenylketonuria but developed normally thanks to an appropriate diet. What forms of variability are associated with his illness and recovery?

CHAPTER V

HEREDITARY PATHOLOGY.

5.1. GENETIC CORRELATION AND ENVIRONMENTAL CONDITIONS IN THE DEVELOPMENT OF PATHOLOGY

The facts accumulated to date by medical genetics allow all the variety of relationships between heredity and environment to be presented in a generalised form.

Let us imagine a situation where the contribution of heredity to the development of a trait, including pathological traits, is zero. This would mean that the trait is completely formed by the external environment, without any participation of the genotype. In other words, the environment would influence "nothing". In fact, the environment always influences one or another material substrate, which is the result of the genes' action. Let us imagine the opposite situation, i.e. when the contribution of heredity is 100%. This would mean that the genetic information about the trait is realised outside the influence of the environment. In reality, the contribution of each of the components to the formation of a trait or property, hence, and disease will be different in different types of pathology.

The organism is a unity of external and internal, an integral system of complexly interrelated parts. Any organism possesses an infinite number of features, although in the empirical description of both healthy and diseased organisms we record only a limited list of properties. Relying on the most general genetic and molecular-biological concepts, it is possible to link many chains of disparate developmental events of both normal and pathological traits. Both normal and pathological traits of an organism are the result of the interaction of hereditary (internal) and environmental (external) factors. That is why a general understanding of pathological processes is possible only by taking into account the results of interaction between heredity and environment. Thus, the genetic programme of an individual in direct or indirect form can participate in the development of pathology.

There are forms of hereditary pathology, the clinical manifestations of which are almost independent of environmental influences. However, this does not mean that everything in man is reduced only to his biology, his genetics. However, today it is quite obvious that outside the phenomenon of heredity no processes of cell life, development of an individual and evolution of organisms are possible.

The fact that human beings are social by nature largely determines the nature of diseases. The increasing share of diseases of non-infectious origin (such as atherosclerosis, CHD, cancer pathology, mental and other diseases) in the structure of morbidity, mortality and disability is almost the most convincing evidence of this. The social nature of man in many respects becomes a determining factor in the realisation of pathological genotypes. Carrying out medical and hygienic measures aimed at preventing the influence of harmful environmental factors, creating conditions conducive to the realisation of normal genotypes and preventing the development of pathological ones, therapy of a number of hereditary diseases are able to reduce the severity of hereditary defects, and in some cases to carry out a complete correction of hereditary disease.

Nowadays, not only microsociety forms specific conditions of genotype realisation. Wide socio-economic transformations significantly change the genetic structure of populations. Changes in population-demographic indicators, such as the level of consanguinity, population density, intensity and direction of migration, marriage system, family size and others, inevitably affect both the spectrum and prevalence of hereditary pathology.

Human socio-economic activity leads to the appearance in the biosphere of new chemical compounds and physical factors with *teratogenic* and *mutagenic* effects.

The scale of environmental pollution by chemical compounds and radiation sources is staggering. Currently, about 7 million artificially created chemical compounds are in the human environment. A resident of a large industrial city comes into contact with almost 50 thousand of them during a day. Despite the lack of rigorous evidence of the relationship between the degree of environmental pollution and the occurrence of genetically determined diseases and congenital anomalies, it can be stated that their number is increasing. Deterioration of the environmental situation may create a background conducive to the realisation of hereditary predisposition to multifactorial diseases. Due to the anthropogenic nature of pathological environmental factors, qualitatively new problems of human gene pool protection arise.

A number of environmental causes can cause diseases in any genotype. Most often this situation is realised in the absence of species protection from environmental agents, but even in this case the nature of the lesion, the scope and diversity of clinical manifestations and other characteristics of the disease are largely determined by the genetic constitution of the organism. On the other hand, even at rigid genetic determination of pathology, environmental conditions, constitutional features, and the whole genotype can have a significant modifying effect on the nature, frequency, and degree of manifestation of a pathological gene. Such high plasticity of genotype creates great opportunities for treatment, prevention of hereditary diseases, development of effective medical and pedagogical programmes of education, rehabilitation and adaptation of patients.

5.2. HEREDITARY CLASSIFICATION

The number of hereditary traits and diseases known to date exceeds more than 10,000, and it is constantly increasing. New, previously unknown hereditary syndromes and diseases are described. Within the framework of already known clinical syndromes, different nosological forms by mechanism of occurrence are distinguished.

Another source of increase in the number of hereditary diseases is the widespread diseases of non-infectious etiology, which include atherosclerosis, hypertension, bronchial asthma, peptic ulcer disease, malignant neoplasms, psoriasis, a number of psychiatric and many other diseases. Modern 109
methods of genetic analysis make it possible to identify monogenic forms among diseases caused by hereditary predisposition, i.e. diseases caused by mutation of a single gene. In this regard, it is necessary to develop a rational classification of hereditary diseases.

The first classifications of hereditary diseases were based mainly on the clinical features of certain groups of pathologies. According to this classification, for example, "hereditary diseases of the skeleton", "hereditary metabolic diseases", "hereditary diseases of the gastrointestinal tract", etc. were distinguished. Since one of the distinguishing features of hereditary disease is the involvement of many organs and systems, the use of a purely clinical (i.e., descriptive) approach does not avoid classification errors. For example, an autosomal dominant hand-heart syndrome, depending on the clinically leading symptom, may be diagnosed as "radial club hand" and, therefore, will be classified within the framework of a purely clinical classification into the group of "skeletal lesions". At the same time, in another patient with an identical mutation (for example, in the brother of the described patient), the leading in the clinical picture of the disease may be a heart lesion with a minimal anomaly of the bone system (in the form of a minor hypoplasia of the thumb). Thus, the second patient falls into the group of hereditary diseases "lesions of the cardiovascular system".

The genetic approach to the classification of inherited diseases is substantial. Such classifications are based on genetic differences, such as the type of mutant cells (either somatic or sexual), or different types of inheritance, etc.

Several classifications of hereditary diseases are currently known.

The classification of hereditary diseases proposed by Academician N.P. Bochkov (1984) is based on the criterion of the specific weight of heredity and environmental influence in the occurrence, developmental features and outcomes of diseases.

Based on this criterion, *four groups of* diseases are distinguished.

Group I - hereditary diseases proper (monogenic and chromosomal). They are caused by mutations. Manifestations of mutations practically do not depend on the environment, i.e. whether there is a disease or not depends only on the presence or absence of mutation. This group of diseases includes, for example, many congenital metabolic disorders: phenylketonuria, mucopolysaccharidoses, galactosemia; disorders of structural protein synthesis: Marfan's disease, osteogenesis imperfecta; hereditary disorders of transport proteins: haemoglobinopathies, Wilson-Konovalov disease; chromosomal diseases: Down's disease, Shereshevski-Turner syndrome, etc.; chromosomal diseases: Down's disease, Shereshevsky-Turner syndrome, etc.

Group II - hereditary diseases caused by mutation, the effect of which is manifested only when the organism is exposed to an environmental factor specific to the mutant gene. This group includes such diseases as hepatic Porphyria, some pharmacogenetic reactions (prolonged respiratory arrest when administering suxamethonium to patients with pseudocholinesterase variant) and ecogenetic diseases (favism).

Group III - diseases, the occurrence of which is largely determined by environmental factors. They unite the majority of widespread diseases, especially diseases of mature and old age. The most frequent and most severe diseases develop in predisposed individuals. Examples of diseases in this group are hypertension, cancer, and mental illness. There is no sharp boundary between groups II and III, and they are often combined into a group of diseases with hereditary predisposition, distinguishing between monotonically or polygenically determined predisposition.

Group IV - diseases caused exclusively by environmental factors (traumas, burns, frostbite, especially dangerous infections, etc.). But even in these diseases genetic factors determine the peculiarities of the clinical course, the effectiveness of therapy, the range of complications, the speed of recovery, the volume of compensatory reactions, the outcome of the disease, etc.

Another widely used classification is based on differences in the primary pathogenetic mechanism of hereditary diseases. From these positions, all hereditary pathology can be divided into *five groups.*

1. ***Genetic diseases*** are diseases caused by gene mutations. They are passed on from generation to generation and are inherited according to Mendel's law.

2. ***Chromosomal diseases*** are diseases resulting from chromosomal and genomic mutations.

3. ***Diseases with hereditary predisposition or multifactorial*** diseases are diseases that arise as a result of a corresponding genetic constitution and the presence of certain environmental factors. Hereditary predisposition is realised by exposure to environmental factors.

4. ***A group of genetic diseases resulting from mutations in somatic cells*** (genetic somatic diseases) has only recently been identified. It includes some tumours, certain malformations, and autoimmune diseases.

5. ***Maternal-fetal genetic incompatibility diseases.*** They develop as a result of an immunological reaction of the mother's body to a foetal antigen.

5.3. PECULIARITIES OF CLINICAL MANIFESTATIONS OF HEREDITARY PATHOLOGY

All diseases (ophthalmological, endocrine, urological, skin, etc.) have their own characteristic features. Similarly, hereditary diseases have their own characteristics, each of which cannot be considered as something absolute. However, when collecting anamnesis, examination, treatment, the presence of these characteristic features in general allows us to suspect hereditary pathology in the patient. The following features are characteristic of hereditary pathology:

1. ***Early manifestation.*** Congenital nature. About 25% of hereditary diseases manifest immediately after birth; about 70% - by three years of life, 90% - by the end of puberty.

2. ***Chronic progressive course.*** A progressive course is a course of the

disease with a constant deterioration of the general condition and an increase in the patient's negative symptoms. The chronic nature of the course of hereditary diseases is determined by the constant functioning of the mutant gene. The degree of chronicity and progression may differ for the same disease.

3. ***Relative resistance to therapy.*** At present it is no longer necessary to speak about absolute resistance to therapy of hereditary diseases. Good results have been achieved in the treatment of certain forms of hereditary pathology. A striking example is phenylketonuria, adrenogenital syndrome, etc.

4. ***Multiplicity of lesions.*** It is known that in more than 60% of hereditary diseases, more than one organ system is involved in the pathological process. For example, in Marfan syndrome, the musculoskeletal system, cardiovascular system and visual organs are affected. Patients with Down syndrome show symptoms of damage to the cardiovascular system, gastrointestinal tract, musculoskeletal system, nervous, respiratory and immune systems.

5. ***Familial nature of the disease.*** If the collection of anamnesis reveals similar cases of the disease in the family, it serves as a direct indication of the hereditary nature of the disease. At the same time, the presence of the disease in only one member of the pedigree does not exclude the hereditary nature of the disease, since the disease may be the result of a new dominant mutation in one of the parents or heterozygosity of both parents for a recessive disease.

6. ***Clinical polymorphism.*** The diversity of clinical and laboratory manifestations of any disease is covered by this concept. For example, some patients with Marfan syndrome can be diagnosed with mitral valve prolapse in the cardiovascular system, and others with aortic aneurysm. On the part of the visual organs, lens subluxation may be noted, mild myopia may be observed, etc.

Every teacher working in preschool education should have concepts about hereditary signs, sinks about - *semiotics.*

Semiotics - the doctrine of signs. Semiotics of hereditary diseases is the doctrine of symptoms of diseases, correct designation of their range, morphological and functional changes of organs and body parts, dynamics of clinical manifestations, i.e. it is a necessary condition for successful diagnosis of the disease.

A huge variety of hereditary diseases, syndromes, malformations are characterised by various combinations of individual signs (symptoms), the total number of which, according to some estimates, exceeds three thousand. According to the clarity of registration, they are subdivided into three groups:

7. *alternative:* either present or absent (examples - preauricular papillomas, cervical fistulae, four-finger palm fold, etc.);
8. *Measuring:* signs defined by absolute or relative quantitative value (lengthening, shortening, enlargement, reduction, etc., examples - arachnodactyly, brachydactyly, macro- and microcephaly, etc.);
9. *descriptive:* signs characterised by changes in skin, hair, soft tissues, etc., to which quantitative assessments are difficult to apply. Unlike the signs of the first group, they require comparative characteristics in their designation (examples - spots on the skin coloured *"coffee and milk",* puckered hair, beak-shaped nose, funnel-shaped chest, etc.).

The pathological phenotype of a certain hereditary syndrome consists of a more or less stable combination of individual symptoms (minimal diagnostic features), which together create a specific "phenotypic core" of the disease, which is the basis for establishing a diagnosis.

Syndrome - a set of external and internal, morphological and functional anomalies and congenital malformations caused by a single morphological factor.

Usually one or another syndrome has from 1-2 to 5 (rarely more) corresponding signs. The task of the educator and doctor is to see these anomalies and interpret them correctly. Such information is important not only for the development of medical treatment and preventive measures, they can and should become the basis for determining the strategy and tactics of psychological and pedagogical correctional work. The difficulty lies in the fact that there is often no parallelism between the significance (in the sense of severity) of a symptom for the patient and its diagnostic value (informativeness) - in the sense of the possibility of establishing a diagnosis.

For example, in the case of Waardenburg syndrome, the main complaint is hearing loss (a variant of congenital neuro-sensory hearing loss due to hypoplasia of the organ of Cortium), and the diagnosis is based on small anomalies found on the scalp and face: grey strand of hair, abnormally short eye slits due to lateral displacement of the inner corners of the eyes (telecanthus), medially expanding eyebrows with a tendency to fuse on the bridge of the nose (sinophrysis), heterochromia of the irises, wide root of the nose. And there are many such examples.

Along with highly informative symptoms in the structure of hereditary syndromes, there are usually background signs: symptoms that are common in many hereditary syndromes (and also in the general population), which together create a background of dysplastic development of the child (*stigmas of dysembryogenesis* are small abnormalities that do not significantly affect the function of the child 114 and do not disfigure the patient's appearance): epicanthus, deformity of the auricles, high palate, altered dermatoglyphics, clinodactyly, various variants of syndactyly, etc.

The diagnostic significance of a single sign of this group is relatively small, but they should not be underestimated, especially when the child has a more serious reason for "claims" in the form of delayed physical, intellectual and sexual development, etc. If two or more (in domestic paediatrics - if 7-10) small anomalies (stigmas of dysembryogenesis) are detected, the patient should undergo a thorough clinical examination.

5.4. PECULIARITIES OF PATHOGENESIS OF MONOGENIC DISEASES

Mutational change of nucleotide sequence of DNA structure is the cause of monogenic hereditary diseases. The specificity of pathogenesis of monogenic diseases is determined by the peculiarities of the chemical nature of the primary product, caused by a particular mutation, and the role that this product plays in the vital activity of the organism. In some mutations, causing the complete absence of a substance necessary for the organism (for example, somatotropic hormone or cytochrome 450), the normal development of the organism is either difficult or impossible; in other mutations, leading to a deficiency of a biologically active substance or structural protein, there are diseases characterised by disorders of the structure and function of individual tissues, organs or physiological systems.

The known variants of the pathogenesis of monogenic diseases are very diverse. This is largely determined by a huge number of violations of biochemical reactions occurring in the body. Despite this, some general regularities of development of monogenic forms of pathology have been identified. For example, for many inherited metabolic diseases (IMDs), a direct link between the mutant gene and the *disturbed biochemical reaction has* been established.

To date, hundreds of types of inherited metabolic anomalies caused by a single mutant gene have been discovered and described in detail. An anomaly of the amino acid sequence of a polypeptide chain caused by a gene mutation significantly disrupts enzyme activity by altering the amount of protein, its information characteristics, thermostability, resistance to various influences, and other properties. In the absolute majority of cases, NDEs are associated with changes in enzyme activity. In turn, mutational disorders of enzyme synthesis lead to disorder or stoppage of reactions in this chain of metabolism, causing the development of one or another form of pathology.

The disease can occur as a result of:

> accumulation of excess substrate as a result of impaired response (e.g. *cerebroside* in Gaucher disease);

> an increase in the content of a precursor substance (e.g. methionine in *cystathioninuria*);

> insufficient substance formation (in particular, cytidine triphosphate deficiency in *orotic aciduria*);

> increased concentration of toxic metabolic products (e.g. phenylacetylglutamine, phenylacetic acid, phenylpyruvic acid and other phenylketone derivatives in *phenylketonuria).*

They are sometimes referred to as gene diseases.

Genetic diseases are a clinically diverse group of diseases caused by mutations of single genes.

The number of currently known monogenic hereditary diseases is about 4000 nosological forms. These diseases occur with an incidence of 1:500-1:100,000 or less.

Different types of mutations occur in the same gene. It is known that the same nosological form can be caused by different mutations. For example, in the cystic fibrosis gene more than 1000 mutations are described, about 300 of which are called clinical manifestations. In the phenylalanine hydroxylase gene, more than 30 mutations cause clinical manifestations of phenylketonuria.

In each gene there can be up to several dozens or even hundreds of mutations leading to diseases. Consequently, it is not difficult to calculate how many monogenic diseases a person could have. In reality, however, a mutational change in the primary structure of a protein often leads to cell death, and the mutation is not realised into an inherited disease. Such proteins are called *monomorphic* proteins. They provide the basic functions of the cell, preserving the stability of its species organisation.

The peculiarities of inheritance of genetic diseases are determined by the laws of H. Mendel (see Chapter H).
Mutations can occur in any genes, leading to disruption (change) of the structure of the corresponding polypeptide chains of protein molecules. Since the human body contains more than 100,000 different types of proteins according to rough estimates, the extreme diversity of clinical manifestations of monogenic diseases becomes understandable. Depending on the function of the altered protein, biochemical changes will occur in the organism, leading to a specific clinical picture of the hereditary disease.
For example, mutations in genes that control the structure of the collagen protein result in generalised connective tissue damage. A mutation in the gene that determines the amino acid sequence of phenylalanine hydroxylase, an enzyme that hydrolyses phenylalanine, results in a disease known as phenylketonuria. Mutations in the globin gene result in a picture of severe anaemia (haemoglobinopathy).
Many gene mutations lead to the formation of such molecular forms of proteins, the pathogenic effect of which is revealed only when the organism interacts with specific environmental factors. These are so-called *ecogenetic variants.* For example, in individuals with clinically not manifested deficiency of glucose-6-phosphate dehydrogenase of erythrocytes, eating horse beans or treatment with oral sulphonamide drugs leads to the development of haemolytic crisis (intravascular decay of erythrocytes). It is important to emphasise that in the absence of contact with certain substances, carriers of "ecogenetic" mutant alleles do not develop pathological reactions or diseases.
The beginning of the pathogenesis of any gene disease is associated with the primary effect of the mutant allele. It can manifest itself in the following variants: absence of protein synthesis, synthesis of protein abnormal in primary structure, quantitatively excessive protein synthesis, quantitatively insufficient protein synthesis.
The principle links in the pathogenesis of gene diseases can be presented as follows: *mutant allele pathological primary product chain of subsequent biochemical reactions cell organs organism.*
Lack of synthesis as a cause of disease development is the most common. A striking example is phenylketonuria, when in the absence of the liver enzyme phenylalanine hydroxylase, phenylalanine cannot be converted to tyrosine. The increased concentration of phenylalanine together with other

toxic substances of its metabolism accumulates in the blood of the patient, affects the developing brain, which leads to the formation of phenylpyruvine oligophrenia.
The same principle of pathogenesis (mutant allele - pathological primary product) applies to morphogenetic control genes, mutations in which lead to congenital malformations (e.g., Holt-Oram syndrome). The onset of birth defect formation is associated with impaired cell differentiation. There are many morphogenetic genes, and they act at different stages of ontogenesis. If the primary product of these genes is abnormal, the cell differentiation necessary for further correct development of the organ does not follow.
For most monogenic diseases, the main link in pathogenesis is the cell. The primary action of the mutant gene is directed at certain cellular structures specific for different diseases (mitochondria, membranes, lysosomes, peroxisomes). Examples of lysosomal diseases are mucopolysaccharidoses, glycogenoses, peroxisomal diseases - Zellweger syndrome, Refsum's disease, mitochondrial diseases - neonatal adrenoleukodystrophy, etc.
A pathological process resulting from a single gene mutation manifests simultaneously at the molecular, cellular and organ levels in any individual.
There are several approaches to the classification of monogenic hereditary diseases: genetic, pathogenetic, clinical and others. The most commonly used classification is based on the *genetic principle.* According to it, monogenic diseases can be subdivided by types of inheritance into: autosomal dominant, autosomal recessive, X-linked dominant, X-linked recessive, U-linked (hollandric) and mitochondrial. This classification is the most convenient, as it immediately allows to orientate about the situation in the family and the prognosis of the offspring.
The second classification is based on the *clinical principle,* i.e. on the assignment of the disease to one or another group depending on the organ system most involved in the pathological process - monogenic diseases of the nervous, respiratory, cardiovascular systems, skin, visual organs, mental, endocrine and so on (see Appendix 2).
The third classification is based on the *pathogenetic principle.* According to it, all monogenic diseases can be divided into hereditary metabolic diseases (hereditary disorders of amino acid metabolism, carbohydrate metabolism disorders, lipid metabolism disorders, steroid metabolism,

etc.), monogenic syndromes of multiple congenital malformations (Halt-Oram syndrome), and monogenic syndromes of multiple congenital malformations (Halt-Oram syndrome)
and combined forms.

The diseases discussed below are the most demonstrative examples from clinical practice arising from gene mutations (enzymeopathies).

5.4.1. AMINO ACID METABOLISM DISEASES

Diseases of amino acid metabolism constitute the largest group of inherited metabolic defects. There are about 60 different forms and, although each of them is rare (1:20,000 to 1:100,000), together they constitute a significant proportion of inherited diseases. Almost all are inherited in an autosomal recessive pattern. Pathogenesis is due to deficiency of one or another enzyme involved in amino acid metabolism. For more than 30 disorders of amino acid metabolism, a specific biochemical defect has been identified as the cause of the disease. Common disorders for this entire group are *aminoaciduria* (excretion of amino acids with urine) and tissue acidosis (disturbance of acid-base equilibrium). It is these homeostasis shifts that cause a number of non-specific clinical symptoms: vomiting and dehydration of the organism, central nervous system dysfunction manifested in soporosis or agitation and convulsions. Later in life, mental retardation is noted.

PHENYLKETONURIA (PHENYLPYRUVINE OLIGOPHRENIA)

Phenylketonuria (PKU) is a disease caused by a congenital defect in amino acid metabolism. This form of the disease was first described by the Norwegian physician F. Fölling in 1934 (in most cases it is called Fölling's disease). Disturbed conversion of phenylalanine to tyrosine leads to accumulation of phenylalanine in the blood, resulting in various pathological phenomena. The incidence in European countries is 1:10,000 newborns.

However, there are significant differences in frequencies between populations. For example, in Turkey it is 1:2,600, in Ireland 1:4,500, in Sweden 1:30,000, and in Japan 1:119,000. PKU is based on a deficiency of phenylalanine hydroxylase, the enzyme that controls the conversion of phenylalanine to tyrosine. As a result of increased phenylalanine concentrations in the body, the formation of the myelin sheath around axons in the central nervous system is impaired.

A newborn with FCU is outwardly normal, but in the first weeks of life it develops clinical signs of neurological pathology: hyperexcitability, increased tendon reflexes, muscle hypertonicity, tremors, convulsive seizures, dyspepsia or, on the contrary, lethargy, drowsiness. Later, with the beginning of feeding in the body begins to enter phenylalanine with mother's milk or with artificial baby food, by 4-5 months of life is noted mental retardation, microcephaly, pale skin, hair, iris. A peculiar "mouse odour" emanates from the sick child.

In children after three years of age, the clinical picture is characterised by mental retardation (in 95% of cases it is imbecility or idiocy), behavioural disorders, and seizure syndrome. It is important to note that the diagnosis of PKU can be made before the appearance of a detailed clinical picture with the help of a simple biochemical test - qualitative determination of phenylpyruvic acid in urine using 3-valent iron chloride.

To avoid false results, the urine is acidified with a few drops of 5% hydrochloric acid solution. The diagnosis is confirmed by determining the serum phenylalanine concentration.

Phenylketonuria is a vivid example of a hereditary disease with a good effect of early preventive treatment, when early diagnosis of the disease and specific dietary therapy (restriction of dairy products) from the first month of a child's life prevents the development of mental retardation, behavioural disorders and other manifestations of the disease.

Dietary therapy is given continuously until puberty with monitoring of blood phenylalanine levels.

ALKAPTONURIA

Alkaptonuria - first described in 1908 by the English physician Archibald Edward Garrod. This disease is inherited in an autosomal recessive manner. Heterozygous carriers of the pathological gene often suffer from arthritis and diseases of the cardiovascular system. The disease occurs in the population with an incidence of 5:1000000.

A newborn with alkaptonuria is outwardly normal, but in the first weeks of life the child shows a dark colour of urine. Later, there is a staining of the sclera and mucous membranes, joints, in the second - third decade develop ochranous arthritis. In alkaptonuria metabolism of phenylalanine and tyrosine is disturbed. Tyrosine obtained with food is normally deaminated to P-hydro- xyphenylpyruvic acid, which is converted to homogentisinic acid. Homogentisine oxidase catalyses the formation of the end products of the breakdown of homogentisic acid.

In alkaptonuria, there is a deficiency of the enzyme homogentisin oxidase in the liver and kidneys. As a result of the enzyme block, large amounts of homogentisic acid accumulate in tissues and physiological fluids.

The disease should be differentiated from rheumatic arthritis if the syndrome is not severe. Treatment, early diagnosis of the disease and specific dietary therapy (with a sharp restriction of phenylalanine and tyrosine) prevents the development of severe forms of arthritis. Large doses of vitamin C are given to improve oxidative processes.

ALBINISM

Albinism is a disease based on an inherited defect in melanin metabolism, resulting in reduced or absent pigment in the skin, mucous membranes, hair, and eyes. In 1660, Baltazar Telles published the History of Ethiopia and gave a description of white Ethiopians. Thus, he is often considered the first to describe an albino (a term derived from the Latin *"albus"* meaning "white"). In fact, Bartolomé Leonardo de Argensola had already described white children born to black parents in New Guinea in his History of the Conquest of the Moluccas Islands in 1609. Argensola is also the first to report the use of the term "albino".

Melanin plays a role in protecting the surface vessels and nuclei of malpighian cells from solar radiation. In this function, it 121
acts as an absorbent that gives off free electrons when exposed to light. Melanin is formed from tyrosine. Depending on whether the synthesis of tyrosinase or other enzymes is impaired, the following clinical forms of albinism are distinguished: ocular-dermal, ocular and cutaneous.

Ocular and cutaneous albinism (albinism type I) - characterised by milky white colouring of the skin and hair. The iris looks transparent grey or blue in oblique light. Pigment in the retina is undetectable, there is no pigmented border of the pupillary margin. The ocular fundus is pale pink in colour. The colour of skin, hair and eyes does not change with age. Photophobia and nystagmus are characteristic. The type of inheritance is autosomal recessive.

Cutaneous albinism is subdivided into albinism without deafness and albinism with deafness. Cutaneous albinism is characterised by congenital depigmented spots with specific localisation: on the head - in the form of a triangle with the base at the eyebrows and the top in the hair area; in the centre of the chin, on the anterior surface of the trunk - from the forearm to the wrist. Ocular symptoms are usually absent; however, there may be iris heterochromia. The type is inherited in an autosomal dominant manner.

Ocular albinism is characterised by the absence of pigment only in the eyes, while in the skin and hair it is present in normal amounts or slightly reduced. The irises are lightly pigmented. Pigmentation of the ocular fundus is so slight that choriodal vessels are visible. With age, pigment accumulates in the iris but not in the retina. Photophobia, nystagmus, and various refractive disorders are observed. The type of inheritance is recessive, X-linked.

5.4.2. CARBOHYDRATE METABOLISM DISEASES

Among them we can distinguish diseases caused by mutations of genes encoding enzymes involved in the breakdown of mono- and disaccharides, e.g. galactosemia, fructosuria, or a group of diseases caused by defects in enzymes involved in the metabolism of polysaccharides, e.g. mucopolysaccharidoses, glycogenoses, etc. These carbohydrates are ingested from food.

The initial symptoms of the disease are seen immediately after birth, as soon as the baby begins to receive milk. The existence of different 122 variants of carbohydrate metabolism diseases and the complexity of biochemical diagnosis make it difficult to recognise these pathologies in a timely manner.

GALACTOSEMIA

Galactosemia - belongs to a group of anomalies of carbohydrate metabolism, which are characterised by lesions of the central nervous system, muscular system, liver dysfunction, erythrocyte abnormalities, hypoglycaemic states.

First described in 1908. Von Reuss. The typical variant of galactosaemia is inherited by autosomal recessive type. The primary biochemical defect in galactosemia is based on a deficiency of galactose-1-phosphate uridyltransferase, resulting in the accumulation of excessive amounts of galactose-1-phosphate and other products of incomplete breakdown of lactose in body tissues, causing clinical manifestations of galactosemia. The incidence is approximately 1:30,000 newborns.

The initial symptoms of the disease are observed immediately after birth, as soon as the baby starts to receive milk. Vomiting, diarrhoea, decreased body weight, jaundice, hepatomegaly (liver changes), bleeding and haemorrhages on the skin occur. Later, cataracts, signs of liver cirrhosis and mental retardation appear. In severe cases, death is possible.

Treatment is pathogenetic. Milk and other products containing galactose are excluded from food. Young children should receive food without galactose: therapeutic milk mixtures devoid of lactose, a mixture of eggs with sugar, rice flour, meat, fish, vegetable purees and broths.

The prognosis is unfavourable in case of late diagnosis and severe forms of the disease. With early dietary treatment, children may develop normally. Patients with milk intolerance should be screened for galactosaemia in the same way as children with a family history of the disease.

MUCOPOLYSACCHARIDOSIS

Mucopolysaccharidoses (MPS) are an example of lysosomal accumulation diseases. Unlike PKU and galactosemia, in which biochemical changes are detected in body fluids, in mucopolysaccharidosis there is intracellular accumulation of products of disturbed catabolism. MPS is a clinically heterogeneous group of hereditary anomalies. Currently, more than 6 variants of this pathology are known. The basis of the pathogenesis of MPS is a violation of the metabolism of acidic glucosaminoglycans, which leads to the deposition of dermatansulfate, chondroitin sulfate and heparan sulfate in the cells of the brain, liver, spleen, bones, kidneys. Rapid diagnosis of MPS is based on qualitative detection of these compounds in urine, good diagnostic results are also obtained by their detection in fibroblast culture. The majority of MPS is inherited by autosomal recessive type; Hunter syndrome is inherited recessively X-linked. Until recently, all MPS were grouped under one general name, *"gargoylism"*.

Mucopolysaccharidosis type I (Hurler syndrome). The disease was first described by Gurler in 1919. It is characterised by severe clinical manifestations, malignant course, leading patients to death at the age of 10-12 years. It is manifested by dwarfism with typical changes in the skull, arms and lumbar spine (lumbar hump) (Fig. 35). Neurological disorders manifest themselves after 4 years of life and are characterised by slowly progressive muscle hypotrophy and hypotonia, seizures, nystagmus, and signs of peripheral neuropathy.

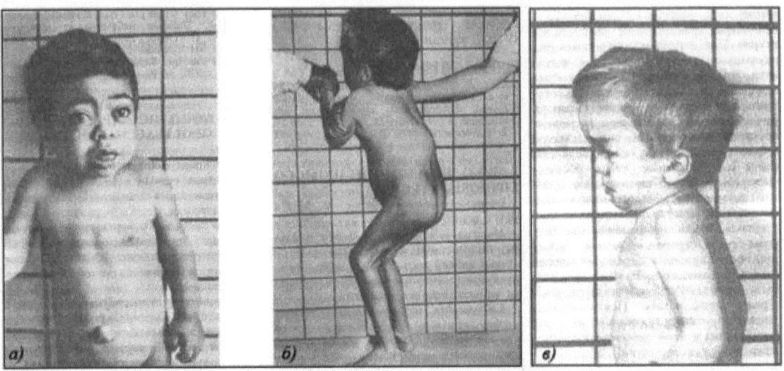

Figure 35. Hurler's syndrome.

a) Tower-shaped skull, coarse facial features (wide nose, thick lips); b) Kyphosis of the spine (curvature of the thoracic or lumbar spine), enlarged abdomen; c) Macro and scaphocephalic skulls.

Mucopolysaccharidosis type II (Gunther syndrome). The disease was described in 1917. S. Gunther. It is characterised by less severe than type I disorders and a somewhat more benign course. Life expectancy of patients on average is about 30 years, in some cases - 60 years. Clinically less pronounced deformities of the skull and limbs, hump is usually absent. Due to the long life expectancy of patients and somewhat less pronounced than in Hurler syndrome, mental retardation and progressive deafness. Patients with type II MPS are noisy and somewhat aggressive. The disease is caused by a recessive mutation of a gene localised in the X chromosome (Fig. 36a).

Mucopolysaccharidosis type III (Sanfillipo syndrome). The disease was first described by S. Sanfillipo in 1963. Clinical signs of the disease are manifested at the age of 3 years and older, increased excitability, inability to concentrate, sometimes aggressiveness. Speech impairment and dementia soon join and progress. There may be deafness, but corneal opacity and other changes in the eyes are not observed. Skeletal changes, joint stiffness slowly increase with age.

There is short stature, shortening of the trunk and upper limbs, short and thickened clavicles. The facial features are coarse (Fig. 366). The life expectancy of patients is up to 20-30 years.

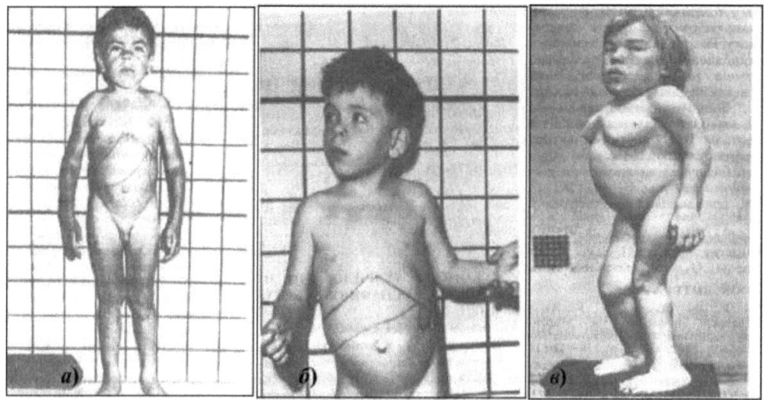

Figure 36. a) Gunther (Hunter) syndrome;
b) Sanfillipo syndrome; c) Marchio and Brailsford syndrome.

Mucopolysaccharidosis type IV (Marchio and Brailsford syndrome). First described in 1929 by L. Marchio and I. Brailsford independently of each other. Clinical signs of the disease appear in the 2nd year of life. Growth retardation begins and skeletal deformities appear (valgus deformity of the knee joints, bulging of the lower ribs, kyphoscoliosis).

The degree of trunk shortening is greater than limb shortening. Intellect is relatively preserved. There is a significant delay in physical development, protruding lower face, hypoplasia of tooth enamel, short neck, scaphocephaly, extremely pronounced lumbar lordosis, large abdomen, and flat feet. Patients have a life expectancy of up to 20 years (Fig. 36c).

5.4.3. LIPID METABOLISM DISEASES

Hereditary defects of lipid metabolism are divided into two groups:

1) Lipidoses or sphingolipidoses are diseases of disturbed catabolism of structural lipids leading to accumulation of sphingolipids in cells of different tissues;

2) diseases with disorders of metabolism of lipoproteins contained in the blood.

Most of these diseases have a similar clinical picture due to impaired catabolism of different but similar sphingolipids. The clinical picture is characterised by progressive dementia, motor disorders, damage to bones, internal organs (liver, spleen, kidneys), skin and retina.

The importance of lipoproteins in the body lies in the transport and distribution of cholesterol and triglycerides to organs. Lipoprotein metabolism is not only under the control of genetic factors, but also

depends to a large extent on nutritional patterns. Therefore, disorders of blood plasma lipid metabolism represent a complex group of conditions, from which only in recent years have monogenically determined defects begun to be distinguished. Hyperlipoproteidaemia is an important factor in the development of atherosclerosis and coronary heart disease.
Most forms of hyperlipoproteidaemia are characterised by early (at the age of 15-20 years) development of atherosclerotic process with clinical picture of angina pectoris, myocardial infarction. Most hyperlipidaemias are inherited by autosomal recessive type.

GANGLIOSIDOSIS

The disease was first described in 1964 by Norman et al. *Gangliosidosis is a* group of diseases caused by defects in lipid metabolism. Currently, 4 types of this pathology are well studied. The common clinical symptoms are: onset of the disease in childhood, symptoms of hypoglycaemia (refusal to eat, vomiting, convulsions, loss of consciousness, coma). Almost all of them are inherited by autosomal recessive type. Pathogenesis is caused by deficiency of one or another enzyme involved in lipid metabolism.

Gangliosidosis type I (Norman-Landing disease). Children with this disease are sharply retarded in psychomotor development from an early age. Pathogenetically, the disease is a defect in the catabolism of gangliosides and insufficiency of P-galactosidase. Patients have a flat nose bridge, hypertelorism, protruding forehead, low-set ears, gingival hypertrophy. Brachydactyly and kyphoscoliosis are found in the skeletal system. Children die at the age of 2-3 years from concomitant bronchopulmonary infections.

Gangliosidosis type II (Tay-Sachs disease or amaurotic idiocy). Children with this syndrome begin to lag in psychomotor development from 4-6 months of age, become apathetic, cease to be interested in their surroundings, stop fixing their gaze. Hyperacusis, muscle hypotonia and blindness due to optic nerve atrophy develop; intelligence declines to the point of idiocy. Gradually complete immobility develops, and convulsions appear. Death usually occurs at 3-4 years of age.

Gangliosidosis type III. The disease was described by Miller et al. in 1974 in a 5-year-old girl. The child developed normally until the age of 5 months. At 5 months of age generalised convulsions appeared, accompanied by increased tendon reflexes, increased tone of the leading leg muscles. Later the convulsions did not recur. The girl began to walk at the age of 2 years, and to speak at the age of 3 years. There were no bone dysplasias during this period, but then there was an enlargement of the medullary cavities of the bones of the arms, ribs, and to a lesser extent - of the bones of the legs. The girl developed microcephaly. Genetic aspects of the disease have not been clarified.

Gangliosidosis type IV. The disease was described by Lauden et al. in 1974. X-ray examinations show thickening of the skull bones, calcification of the basal ganglia, osteoporosis of the long tubular bones, and posture disorders. The patient at the age of 4-5 years shows some awkwardness of movements. Then regression of mental and motor functions is noted, speech and purposeful activity are lost.

Leukodystrophy. A group of inherited diseases of the nervous system characterised by progressive decay of the white matter of brain tissue (dysmyelination) due to a defect in enzymes involved in lipid catabolism and myelin synthesis. The brain is affected diffusely, with both hemispheres, brain stem, and cerebellum affected symmetrically. The disease is described in three clinical variants, differing in the time of appearance of the first symptoms and the rate of course: early infantile form, infantile and late infantile form.

5.5. PECULIARITIES OF PATHOGENESIS OF CHROMOSOMAL DISEASES

A characteristic feature of the pathogenesis of chromosomal diseases is an early disorder of morphogenesis. It is manifested by a disorder of cell division and maturation, impaired cell migration and differentiation, which causes the formation of multiple malformations of various organs and tissues. The observed phenomena are believed to be based on genome imbalance.

There are three types of effects in the development of chromosomal diseases: specific, semi-specific and non-specific. *Specific* effects are associated with changes in the number of structural genes encoding protein synthesis (unique for any chromosome). In trisomies the number of them increases, in monosomies it decreases. *Semi-specific* effects in chromosomal diseases are caused by changes in the number of genes represented in the genome by a large number of copies (for example, genes of ribosomal, histone, contractile proteins, etc.). *Non-specific* manifestations of chromosomal aberrations can be caused by changes in the content of heterochromatin, which fulfils an important role in the processes of cell division, growth, etc. In chromosomal aberrations, the severity of deviation from normal development, as a rule, correlates with the degree of chromosomal imbalance. The more chromosomal material involved in the aberration, the earlier the disease will manifest itself in ontogenesis and the more significant the disorders in the physical and mental development of the individual. An excess of chromosomal material is less clinically significant than its loss.

For example, the loss of one of the autosomal chromosomes prevents implantation of the egg in the uterus. At the same time, chromosomal syndromes due to trisomies on different chromosomes are known. The excess or deficiency of heterochromatised regions of chromosomes may not have clinical consequences. In contrast, loss of euchromatin always results in the loss of unique genes.

5.6. CHROMOSOMAL DISEASES

Chromosomal diseases are a large group of congenital inherited diseases that are clinically characterised by the presence of multiple malformations and have numerical or structural abnormalities of chromosomes as their etiological basis. Clinicians began studying chromosomal diseases even before the exact number of human chromosomes was established. For example, Klinefelter and Sherechevsky-Turner syndromes were clearly described before the discovery of the chromosomal etiology of these diseases and are well known to clinicians.

All chromosomal diseases can be divided into three groups:

1) complete forms with a change in the number of chromosomes;
2) complete forms with a change in chromosome structure;
3) mosaic forms with chromosomal or genomic mutations.

Many human chromosomal anomalies have already been described. According to the data given in the monograph by N.P. Bochkov, chromosomal anomalies of gametic origin alone number about 750, of which the share of structural rearrangements accounts for more than 700.

Numerical changes of chromosomes are reduced to the presence of additional chromosomes or the absence of one of the chromosomes. In the first case we speak of trisomy on any of the 23 chromosomes, in the second case - monosomy. Less often, one can observe a violation of the ploidy of the chromosome set (increase by a full haploid set). Such genomic mutations are most often found in spontaneous abortus and can be represented by triploidy and tetraploidy. Phenotypically, these individuals are female with delayed growth and sexual development, normal external and underdeveloped internal genitalia.

Structural changes in human chromosomes, although much less frequent than numerical aberrations, are of interest both theoretically and clinically. Two main types of rearrangements can be distinguished: *intrachromosomal* and *interchromosomal* (see 4.1.2.).

Most chromosomal diseases occur sporadically as a result of genomic and chromosomal mutations in the gametes of healthy parents or in the first divisions of the zygote. Chromosomal changes in gametes lead to the development of the so-called complete, or regular, forms of karyotype disorders, and the corresponding changes in chromosomes at early stages of embryo development are the cause of somatic *mosaicism*, or *mosaic organisms* (the presence in the organism of two or more cell lines with different numbers of chromosomes).

Mosaicism can involve both sex chromosomes and autosomes. Mosaics tend to have more "erased" forms of the disease than people with an altered number of chromosomes in each cell. Thus, a child with a mosaic variant of Down's disease may have normal intelligence, but the physical signs of the disease remain.

The number of abnormal cells may vary: the more there are, the more pronounced is the symptom complex of a particular chromosomal disease. In some cases, the specific weight of abnormal cells is so small that the person seems phenotypically healthy. Chromosomal anomalies have a wide range of clinical manifestations. They can cause congenital malformations, repeated spontaneous abortions, stillbirths, neonatal mortality and infertility.

A definitive diagnosis of chromosomal pathology is possible only after cytogenetic analysis (karyotyping). The nurse and laboratory assistant, together with the doctor, should know the forms for recording both normal and abnormal karyotypes (see Appendix 3). Preschool teachers should also have a general understanding of karyotype records.

5.7. AUTOSOMAL TRISOMIES

DOWN SYNDROME (DOWN'S DISEASE)

The first clinical description of this anomaly dates back to 1866 and belongs to the English physician Langton Down. To date, Down's disease has been studied quite comprehensively, as it is one of the most frequent chromosomal diseases. The frequency of this syndrome among newborns is 1:700-800.

In the vast majority of cases (up to 94%), simple trisomy 21 is found in patients. About 4% of cases are due to translocation form of trisomy with involvement of other acrocentric chromosomes and in 2% of cases mosaicism is detected.

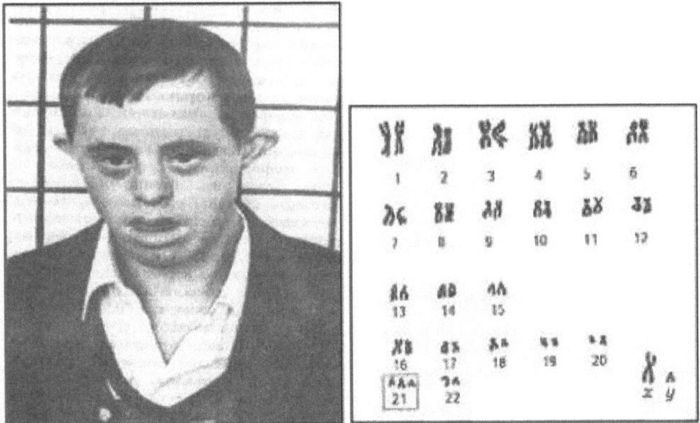

Figure 37. Down syndrome. (47, HU, +21).

Down's disease affects girls and boys at the same rate. The frequency of birth is not affected by racial, geographical or population differences, but there is a correlation between the birth of these patients and the age of the mother. The older the mother, the greater the risk of having a child with Down's disease. Mothers aged 40-44 have a 16 times higher risk of having an abnormal offspring than mothers aged 20-24. Down syndrome patients are usually short in stature, characterised by dementia and numerous physical malformations (Figure 37).

They have a characteristic appearance and are very similar to each other in many respects. Diagnosis of the disease is not difficult for obstetricians and paediatricians, even in patients of different ethnic groups. Characteristic features: a small round head with a slanted back of the head, slanted eye slits, short nose with a wide flat nose bridge, small deformed ears, half-open mouth with a protruding tongue and protruding lower jaw, peculiar gait with awkward movements, eloquence. In the 1st year of life, children with Down's disease are noticeably behind in motor and mental development. They start sitting and walking later, their muscles are sharply hypotonic, the volume of movement is increased in the joints.

Cardiovascular malformations are particularly common in children with Down's disease, and gastrointestinal malformations are sometimes observed. Much less common are kidney and urinary tract malformations, as well as hearing impairment. Of the characteristic dermatoglyphic features of Down's disease, let us mention two:

1) "monkey fold" - a deep transverse furrow; 2) a single flexor fold on the little finger, quite often symmetrical on both hands.

Due to continuous improvements in medical care, the life expectancy of patients with Down syndrome has increased significantly. Whereas previously such patients died in early childhood from various infectious diseases, now they live up to 30 years and more. Treatment is mainly symptomatic.

Stimulating therapy (vitamins, hormones, etc.) is widely used. Medical, pedagogical and therapeutic measures make it possible to adapt some patients to feasible labour activity.

PATAU SYNDROME (TRISOMY 13)

According to numerous generalisations, the incidence of Patau syndrome, described in 1960, ranges from 1:700-8000. As in Down's disease, children with Patau syndrome are more likely to be born to older mothers. The frequency of the syndrome is similar among both sexes. At the heart of Patau syndrome is non-disjunction on the 13th pair of chromosomes. There are 47 chromosomes with an extra chromosome 13 in the patient's karyotype.

The appearance of patients with Patau syndrome is very specific. Sick newborns are normal in size and weight (Fig. 38a; b; c).

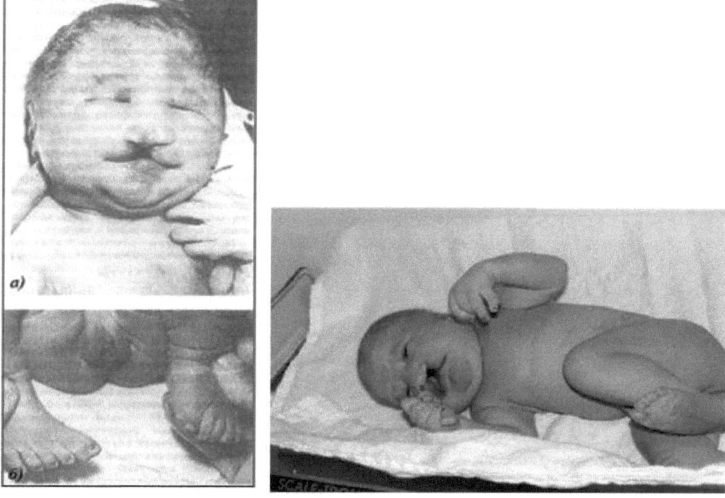

Figure 38. Patau syndrome.

a) facial anomalies; b) bilateral polysyndactyly of the feet; c) a newborn child with cleft lip and palate.

Clinical features include severe mental retardation, pronounced microcephaly, malformed and low-set ears, eyeball anomalies (microphthalmia and anophthalmia), uni- or bilateral lip and palate malformation, polydactyly, increased joint flexibility, congenital malformations of internal organs, and seizures are often observed. Deafness in patients with trisomy 13 occurs in 80-85% of cases.

Pathological examination reveals multiple external and internal deformities of almost all organs and systems. Brain mass is reduced, sometimes the brain is not divided into hemispheres. Heart defects, anomalies of the kidneys, ureters (doubling) and gastrointestinal tract are often found. On the basis of clinical, dermatoglyphic and pathological anatomical data, the diagnosis is not difficult to make. It is finally confirmed cytogenetically. The prognosis in Patau syndrome is unfavourable, and there are no successful treatment methods.

EDWARDS SYNDROME (TRISOMY 18)

The syndrome was described in 1960. The syndrome was described in I960 by D. Edwards and was subsequently named after him. The frequency of Edwards syndrome among newborns is 1:7000. Girls are affected about 3 times more often. The reasons for the predominance of girls are still unclear. Trisomy 18 in almost all cases is a consequence of non-disjunction of the 18-pair of chromosomes, usually at the stage of meiosis, sometimes at the stage of zygote (mosaicism), translocation forms are very rare. Children with this syndrome are born with low birth weight.

a)

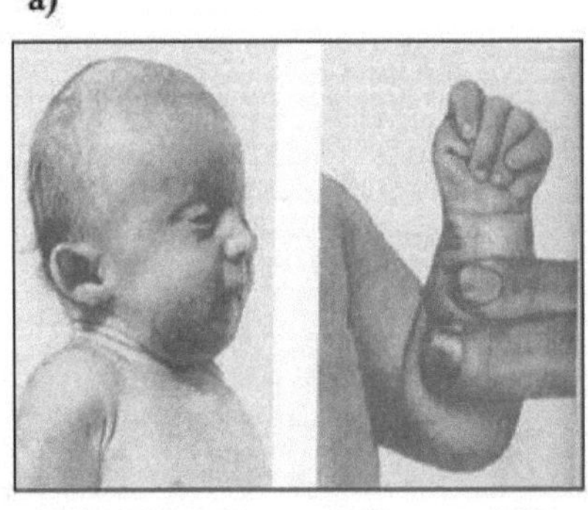

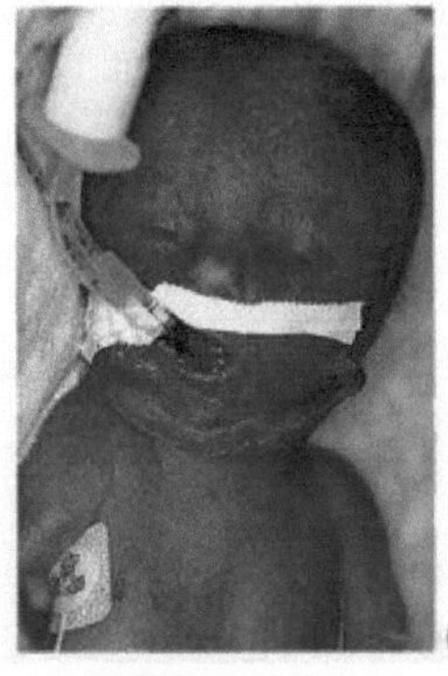

б)

Figure 39. Edwards syndrome, a) auricles low, rotated backwards, eye slits narrow *and* short, mandible *and* mouth opening small; b) flexor position of hands.

The phenotypic manifestations of Edwards syndrome are quite characteristic: the skull is dolichocephalic, the mandible and mouth opening are small, the eye slits are narrow and short, the auricles are small and low, the external ear canal is narrowed, sometimes absent (Fig. 39a; b). The sternum is short, the thorax is broad. The flexor position of the hands is characteristic, sometimes there is aplasia of the thumb and radial bones, and a "rocking foot" is noted. Of the external signs should be mentioned spinal hernias, and cleft lip. Of the malformations of internal organs are the most constant malformations of the heart and large vessels, gastrointestinal tract, incomplete turn of the intestine, atresia of the gallbladder and biliary tract. On the side of the central nervous system, hypoplasia and aplasia of the corpus callosum and hypoplasia of the cerebellum are most often noted. Malformations of the urinary system and genital organs.

Life expectancy in children with Edwards syndrome is sharply reduced - 60% of patients die before the age of 3 months. One child out of 10 survives to a year. In the mosaic form, life expectancy is much higher. But all surviving children have profound idiocy.

CATCALL SYNDROME

The "cat cry" syndrome was first described by J. Lejeune in 1963 in 3 children with multiple anomalies, profound mental retardation and characteristic crying that resembled a cat cry. Currently, more than 300 children with this peculiar syndrome have been identified. Cytologically, all patients show a shortening of the

approximately one-third of the short arm of one of the homologues of chromosome 5. The incidence of this disease is not precisely known, but is approximately 1:45,000 with a male to female sex ratio of 1:1.3.

The clinical syndrome of "catcall" is highly polymorphic.

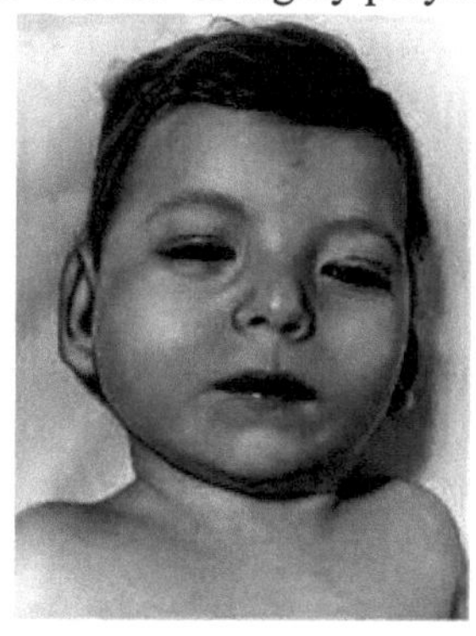

Figure 40. The "cat-cry" syndrome.

Without a peculiar cry in the patient, it is impossible to establish a reliable diagnosis before cytological examination, since most of the clinical symptoms of this disease are also found in other chromosomal anomalies. The occurrence of specific crying is associated with changes in the larynx - narrowing, softness of the cartilage, swelling or unusual folding of the mucosa, and reduction of the epiglottis. These children are also often diagnosed with microcephaly, low and deformed auricles, microgenia, moon-shaped face, hypertelorism, antimongoloid eye shape, strabismus, and muscular hypotonia (Figure 40). Children are dramatically retarded in physical and mental development. Diagnostic signs such as "cat cry", moon-shaped face and muscle hypotonia disappear completely with age, while microcephaly, on the contrary, becomes more pronounced, and mental retardation progresses. Life expectancy of patients is short, there is no treatment.

5.8. SEX CHROMOSOME ABNORMALITIES

Sex chromosome abnormalities in humans are most commonly trisomies and monosomies. Both types of anomalies occur when two types of gametes, normal and pathological (with or without an extra sex chromosome), fuse. These anomalies are caused by chromosome divergence, either during one or two meiosis divisions during gametogenesis in one of the parents, or during early mitotic divisions of the zygote.

The cumulative frequency of chromosomal anomalies on sex chromosomes is 2.6 per 1000 births, which is slightly less than theoretical. The data obtained indicate the selective death of zygotes at the foetal stage and children of 5 years of age with a violation of the number of sex chromosomes. In women, the most frequent sex chromosome abnormalities are the Shereshevsky-Turner (XO) and trisomy-X (XXX) syndromes, and in men - the Klinefelter syndrome (XXX) and double chromosome U (XXX).

SCHERESCHEWSKY-TURNER SYNDROME

The clinical picture of this syndrome was first described by N.A. Shereshevsky in 1925. A classic but more complete description belongs to Henry Turner (1938). Cytogenetically, the syndrome (XO) was discovered by Ford in 1959. Further studies showed that in Shereshevski-Turner syndrome, the cells of the organism lack sex chromatin and have only one X chromosome.

The frequency of the syndrome among newborn girls is 1:2000 to 1:5000. About 95% of zygotes with a chromosome set (CS) die intrauterine. Patients with Shereshevsky-Turner syndrome are of short stature (Fig. 41) and have a peculiar thyroid chest and widely spaced nipples.

They are very often observed. Wing-like folds on the neck, deformed ear flaps, valgus deformity of the elbows, many birthmarks on the skin. The face of patients is very similar to the face of the "sphinx" because of the reduced chin, wide nose bridge and hypertelorism, epicanthus, ptosis.

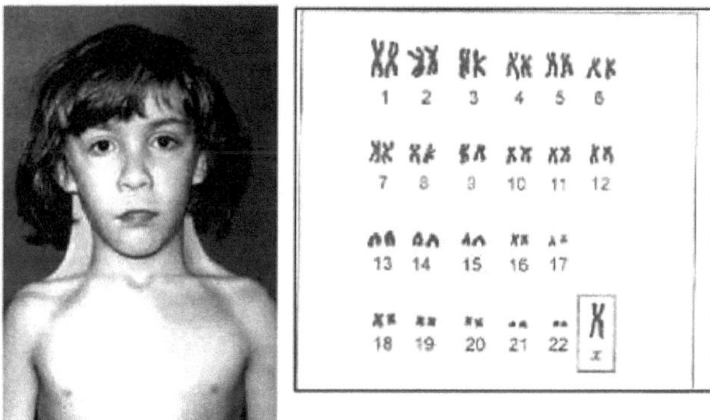

Figure 41. Shereshevsky-Turner syndrome.

In this syndrome, there is dysgenesis of the gonads, increased urinary gonadotropin levels, primary amenorrhoea, infertility, and underdevelopment of secondary sexual characteristics. In 50% of cases, the patients are mentally retarded. They are passive, and prone to psychogenic reactions. The preliminary diagnosis of this syndrome is based on the characteristic clinical picture and the study of sex chromatin, the final diagnosis is based on the results of cytogenetic analysis. Treatment is mainly symptomatic and is usually aimed at the correction of secondary sexual characteristics.

TRISOMY "X" SYNDROME

The syndrome of trisomy on chromosome X was first described by Jacobson in 1959. Its incidence is 1:1000 to 1:2000 newborn girls.

The clinical picture of this disease is extremely diverse. As a rule, physical and mental development in women with this syndrome has no deviations from the norm.

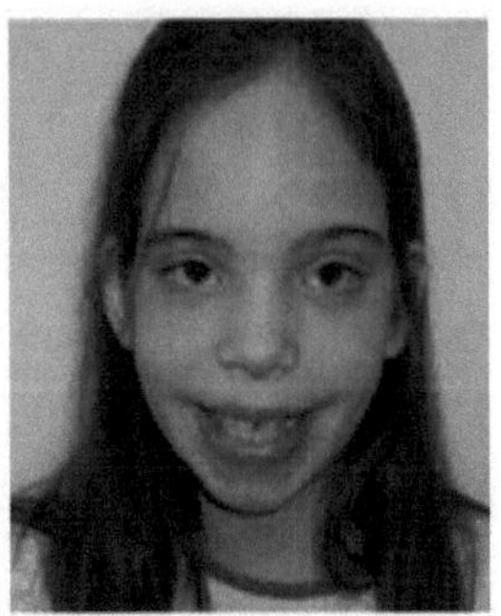

Figure 42. Trisomy X syndrome.

This is because two X chromosomes are inactivated and one continues to function as in normal women. Changes in the karyotype are usually detected incidentally during an examination.

Mental development is also usually normal, sometimes at the lower limits of normal. Only in some women

reproductive disorders (various cycle disorders, secondary amenorrhoea, early menopause). In X trisomies, there is a high growth of the male physique, epicanthus, hypertelorism, flattened nose bridge, high palate, abnormal growth of teeth, deformed and abnormally located auricles (Fig. 42), clinodactyly of little fingers, transverse palm fold. It is proved that among them one can find persons with psychopathic traits and inclination to schizophrenic-like disorders several times more often. Many studies have noted a peculiar feature: as the number of X chromosomes in the karyotype increases to 4; 5 and more, the clinical manifestations of the syndrome increase.

Patients with 4 or 5 X chromosomes are mentally more retarded and, as a rule, their generative function is severely impaired. Treatment is mainly symptomatic and aimed at correcting the endocrine imbalance.

KLEINFELTER SYNDROME

The clinic of Klinefelter syndrome was described in 1942 by G.F.Klinefelter, in 1956 P.Jacobs and J.Strong confirmed the chromosomal etiology of this disease (47, XXU).

Klinefelter syndrome occurs in 1:500 to 700 newborn boys. Several types of X and U chromosome polysomy have been found in males: 47, XXU; 48, XXXU; 49, XXXU; 47, XUU; 48, XUU, etc. The diagnosis cannot be suspected during the newborn period. The main clinical manifestations manifest during puberty.

Men with Klinefelter syndrome are characterised by tall stature, long limbs, eunuchoidism, impaired spermatogenesis resulting in infertility, gynaecomastia, shrunken testes, increased secretion of female sex hormones, a tendency to obesity, and scanty hair in the axillae (Fig. 43). Patients with this syndrome are highly suggestible, lethargic, apathetic, uninitiative, and often have mental retardation (usually debility). Paranoid, depressive psychoses are not uncommon.

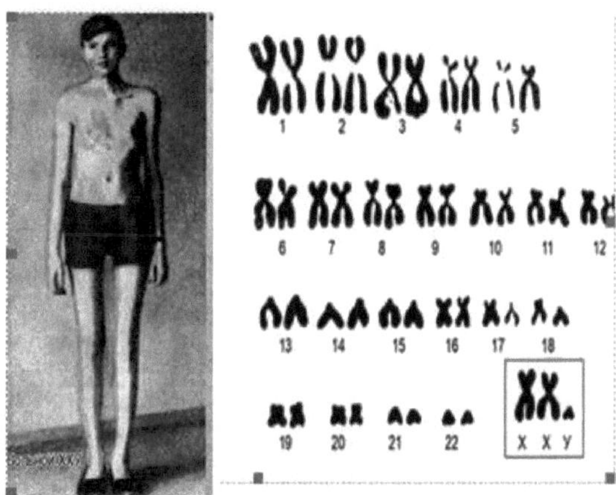

Figure 43. Klinefelter's syndrome.

Klinefelter syndrome is not difficult to diagnose, especially in adults. The peculiar combination of tall stature, female skeletal structure, gynaecomastia, obesity and decreased intelligence suggests Klinefelter syndrome even without sex chromatin testing.

Treatment with testosterone and methyltestosterone is aimed at correcting secondary sexual characteristics. However, patients remain infertile even after therapy.

Y-CHROMOSOME DISOMY SYNDROME

This syndrome was first described in 1961 by A. Sandberg et al. and defined its cytogenetics - 47, HUU.

The frequency of this syndrome among newborn boys is 1:840 and increases to 10% in tall males (above 200 cm).

Most patients have accelerated growth during childhood. The average height of adult males is 186 cm. In most cases, they do not differ from normal individuals in physical and mental development. There are no noticeable abnormalities in the sexual and endocrine systems, as well as in fertility. Although some peculiarities of behaviour in such persons are not excluded - they are prone to aggressive and criminal acts.

About 30-40% of patients have certain symptoms - coarse facial features, protruding brow arches and bridge of the nose, enlarged lower jaw, high palate, abnormal growth of teeth with defects of tooth enamel, large auricles, pathology of knee and elbow joints. Sometimes there are various disorders of the sexual sphere, borderline mental retardation or mild debility. Life expectancy in such patients does not differ from the population.

5.9. MULTIFACTORIAL INHERITANCE

The gene and chromosomal diseases discussed in the previous sections are entirely determined by pathological heredity, i.e. mutations. At the same time, a wide range of diseases are known, such as hypertension, some forms of diabetes mellitus, bronchial asthma, peptic ulcer disease, atherosclerosis, schizophrenia, congenital malformations and many others, the occurrence of which largely depends on environmental factors.

The emergence of widespread diseases that contribute most to morbidity, disability and mortality is determined by the interaction of ***hereditary factors*** and a variety of ***environmental factors.*** This ***multifaceted*** group of diseases is called diseases with hereditary predisposition or ***multifactorial pathology.*** Hereditary predisposition to diseases is based on the great genetic diversity (genetic polymorphism) of human populations in enzymes, structural, transport proteins and antigenic systems.

Multifactorial diseases (MFDs), for all their diversity, are characterised by some common features:

1) high frequency in the population;
2) wide clinical polymorphism (from latent subclinical to severe manifestations);
3) significant age and sex differences in the frequency of individual forms;
4) earlier onset and some intensification of clinical manifestations in descending generations;
5) relatively low level of concordance on manefest manifestations of the disease in monozygotic twins (60% and below), however, significantly increased corresponding level in dizygotic twins;
6) inconsistency of the pattern of inheritance with simple Mendelian models;
7) similarity of clinical manifestations in the patient and his immediate family members;
8) dependence of the degree of disease risk for healthy relatives on the general frequency of the disease, the number of sick relatives in the

family, the severity of the course of the disease in the sick relative, etc.
Hereditary predisposition to various diseases may have a different genetic basis. In some cases, hereditary predisposition is determined by a single mutant gene, in others it is formed by the combined action of several genes. In the first case, we speak of a monogenic predisposition, in the second case - the polygenic basis of the disease.
Monogenic diseases with hereditary predisposition are characterised by the fact that the predisposition to the development of the disease is determined by only *one mutant gene.* For the pathological manifestation of the mutant gene requires a mandatory action, usually a specific external environmental factor. Such effects may be associated with physical, chemical, including drugs, drugs and biological factors. Without the influence of a specific factor, even in the presence of a mutant gene in the genotype, the disease does not develop. If an individual does not have such a mutation, but is exposed to a specific environmental factor, the disease does not develop. To date, more than 40 genes are known, mutations in which can cause disease under the action of "manifesting" environmental factors specific to each gene.
Polygenic diseases with hereditary predisposition are determined by the combination of alleles of several genes. Any one of the genes included in the "predisposition complex" usually has a small but summative effect on the formation of predisposition. Geneticists call such an influence *additive (additive).* In practice, there are significant difficulties in differentiating situations when the disease is caused only by the polymeric nature of gene interaction or by a combination of the interaction of several genes and environmental factors (multifactorial diseases).
Multifactorial traits may be *discontinuous* or *continuous,* but any such disease is always determined by the interaction of gene and environmental factors. In medicine, a number of anomalies and various diseases are known for which it is assumed that they occur in individuals with a multifactorial predisposition that increases some defect. Let us give examples of some intermittent MFB human diseases:

- isolated congenital malformations: cleft lip and palate, congenital heart defects, neural tube defects, pylorostenosis;
- frequent diseases in adults: hypertension, rheumatoid arthritis, peptic ulcer disease, schizophrenia, epilepsy, bronchial asthma.

For these and similar pathological conditions, a higher frequency in close relatives compared to the general population, the dependence of the risk of disease development on the degree of kinship with the diseased person and the severity of the proband's disease are noted. As a rule, there is no distribution of sick and healthy people in the pedigrees of probands characteristic for monogenic diseases.

Control Questions and Assignments:

1. Which pathology is called hereditary?
2. Into which groups can all hereditary diseases be divided?
3. Give a brief characterisation of gene-based diseases?
4. How do genetic diseases arise?
5. What type of amino acid metabolism disease is inherited?
6. Give a brief characterisation of the clinical manifestations of amino acid metabolism disease?
7. At what frequency are babies born with phenylketonuria?
8. List the diseases arising from disorders of carbohydrate metabolism?
9. At what age intervals is the risk of having children with chromosomal abnormalities dramatically increased?
10. What are the causes of trisomies?

TEST-5.

1. What is the name of the trait hexapalatia. The degree of severity of the trait can vary greatly. There may be six fingers on all limbs or only on one, two, or three limbs. Sometimes there are seven toes. It is inherited in an autosomal dominant pattern.

a) polydactyly.
б) syndactyly.
(c) Brachydactyly.
e) arachnodactyly.

2. What is the name of a disease characterised by disproportionately short limbs with a normally developed torso, dwarfism, and a nose often saddle-shaped. The vast majority of children die intrauterine, born viable. It is inherited as a dominant autosomal trait.

a) Vitiligo;
б) Arachnodactyly;
в) Achondroplasia;
e) Alkaptonuria

3. What is the name of a disease characterised by non-clotting of blood. It is associated with the absence of various clotting factors involved in the formation of plasma thromboplastin. It is inherited as a recessive, sex-linked trait.

a) Haemophilia.
б) Alkaptonuria.
(c) Galactosemia.
e) Cystonuria.
4. Which patients have tall stature, asthenic physique and arm span exceeding height, characterised by a combination of various skeletal, ocular and visceral anomalies: long and thin limbs with very long and thin fingers, lens dislocation, aortic aneurysm, urinary excretion of certain amino acids, asthenic constitution. Autosomal dominant inheritance with a penetrance of 30%.
a) Shereshevsky-Turner syndrome.
б) hand-heart syndrome;
(c) Klinefelter syndrome;
e) Marfan syndrome;
5. In which syndrome are "coffee and milk" type pigments observed.
a) Neurofibromatosis; b) Albinism; c) Vitiligo; e) Alkaptonuria.

CHALLENGE-5.

1. According to the anamnesis, the mother is healthy and comes from a family favourable for one of the forms of ichthyosis (X-linked recessive inheritance type), and the father has this form of ichthyosis. The daughter of these parents marries a healthy young man. Determine the genetic risk of having a child with this form of ichthyosis in this young family.
What prenatal diagnostic methods can be used to detect this disease in the foetus? What recommendations should be made by a geneticist?
2. Phenylketonuria is inherited as a recessive trait. What can children in a family where the parents are heterozygous for this trait be like?
3. In some people, erythrocyte antigens (*A* and *B*) may be present in saliva. The presence of *A* and *B* antigens in saliva is determined by gene *S* - secretors, gene *s* - non-secretors. During the study of blood and saliva of 4 family members it was found that the mother has antigen *B* in erythrocytes, but does not contain it in saliva; the father contains antigen *A* in both erythrocytes and saliva; in the erythrocytes of the first child there are antigens *A and B*, but they are not in saliva; in the second child there are no antigens *A and B* in both erythrocytes *and* saliva. Determine the genotypes of all of these individuals, if possible.
4. In humans, brown eye colour dominates blue eye colour and dark hair colour dominates light hair colour. The genes for both traits are in different pairs of chromosomes. A blue-eyed, dark-haired father and a brown-eyed,

light-haired mother have four children, each of whom differs from each other in these traits. Determine the genotypes of the parents.

5. A healthy woman whose brother has haemophilia married a healthy man. During differential diagnosis of the brother's disease, haemophilia *B*, inherited as a sex-linked recessive trait, was diagnosed, which was confirmed by pedigree analysis. The penetrance of haemophilia *B* is 100%. Define:

а) the likelihood that the first child will be sick;

б) the probability that if there are two children in a family, one of them will be sick.

CHAPTER VI

HEREDITARY FORMS OF MENTAL AND PHYSICAL DEVELOPMENTAL DISORDERS

For many decades, the leading factors in the etiology of persistent deviations in mental and physical development were considered to be perinatal hazards, pathology of childbirth, traumas, infections, and intoxications of early age. Advances in medical and biological sciences have led to a radical revision of these ideas. Over the years, many hereditary diseases and syndromes have been discovered, and it is now reasonably believed that among persistent disorders of mental and physical development are often hereditary forms.

The identification of hereditary forms is not only of considerable theoretical interest, but is also of great practical importance. If the hereditary aetiology of a developmental disorder is definitely established, this first of all makes it possible to draw up more accurate and complete ideas about its clinical picture (for example, about the most probable complicating symptoms and syndromes), about possible variants of dynamics and prognosis. Such information is important not only for the development of medical treatment and preventive measures, they can and should become the basis for determining the strategy and tactics of psychological and pedagogical correctional work. In addition, there is an opportunity to develop scientifically based criteria for medical and genetic counselling and family planning.

Mental retardation (the term "Intellectual disability" is often used as a synonym) is not a purely clinical concept, but a medical and pedagogical one. Mental retardation is a persistent impairment of cognitive activity due to brain damage. Mental retardation is heterogeneous by many parameters - etiology, clinical picture, dynamics, clinical and psychological structure of the defect, etc.

The majority of mentally retarded children (75-80%) suffer from oligophrenia. This is a group of morbid conditions, the clinical picture of which is characterised by:

- phenomena of general (not only intellectual or mental) underdevelopment;
- the prevalence of abstract thinking deficiency in the structure of intellectual defect;
- lack of progression, evolutionary nature of dynamics;

- Early, before 2-2.5 years of age (i.e., in the pre-speech period), onset.

Dementia occurs at a later age than oligophrenia, and its causes can be very different (exogenous organic brain damage, unfavourable schizophrenia and epilepsy, some hereditary degenerative diseases).

The clinical picture of dementia (unlike oligophrenia) is dominated by the phenomena of damage, disturbance, disintegration of already formed (at least partially) functions, while signs of underdevelopment, if they occur, do not dominate the clinical picture. The dynamics of dementia in the remote period (the most important for correctional pedagogy) can be very different - from evolutionary to pronounced progredient.

It is quite understandable that unambiguous differentiation between dementia and oligophrenia is not always possible and is especially difficult at the age of 2-4 years, when the signs of underdevelopment and damage are quite correlated in their contribution to the structure of clinical manifestations. Nevertheless, the distinction between oligophrenia and dementia is desirable even from a purely practical point of view, since each of these types of mental retardation requires a specific strategy of corrective measures and may differ in prognosis.

As we have already mentioned, for a long time it was believed that early (up to 2-2.5 years of age) non-progressive forms of mental retardation, i.e. oligophrenia, were mainly exogenously caused pathology. In the last 25-30 years this position has been radically revised, and according to the data of both domestic and foreign scientists, /$^3_4$ cases of mental retardation are genetically determined and only % is associated with exogenous causes.

It should be emphasised that mental retardation in hereditary diseases is usually one of the symptoms in a complex clinical picture of the disease. For some hereditary diseases, mental retardation is an obligatory symptom, while in some other hereditary diseases it is not observed in all cases.

Depending on the nature of the genetic disorder, a distinction is made:

1) mental retardation in chromosomal diseases;
2) mental retardation in monogenic diseases;
3) multifactorial mental retardation.

6.1. MENTAL RETARDATION IN CHROMOSOMAL DISEASES

The frequency of chromosomal diseases among newborns is 0.50.7 per cent, and 2.2 per cent among stillborns and children who died before one year of age. Oligophrenia due to various chromosomal disorders accounts for about 10-12% of all cases of mental retardation.

The main clinical feature of chromosomal diseases is mental retardation and multiple malformations. Among children with multiple malformations, chromosomal diseases are registered in 42.6% of cases.

Among quantitative autosomal disorders, ***Down syndrome*** is the most frequent and therefore the most well-known (Fig. 44). At present, children with this pathology account for up to 10% of the pupils of special schools of the VIII kind. All Down syndrome patients suffer from intellectual disability: 5% - mild, 75% - moderate and pronounced, 20% - profound.

The main feature of the psychopathological status is general mental underdevelopment. Thinking is stiff, sluggish, children are incapable of abstraction. Temporal relations are more difficult to establish than spatial ones.

If children with Down syndrome master abstract numeracy, they do so with great difficulty. Reading is easier than writing; many read fluently and even expressively (imitating adult voice modulations).

Retelling only by questions, independent retelling is very difficult or inaccessible.

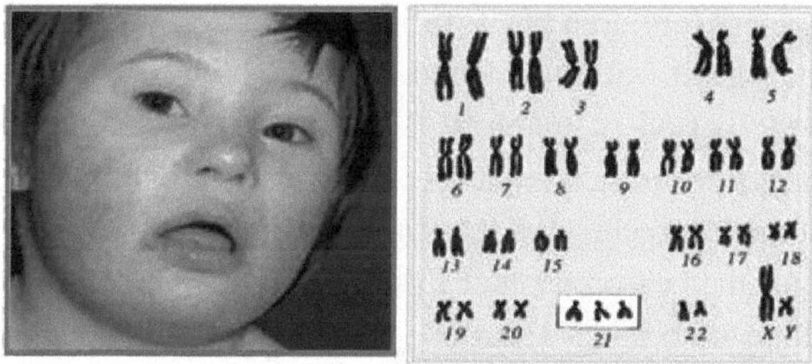

Figure 44. Down syndrome.

Speech develops late: the first words typically appear by the age of five, and simple phrases by the age of eight. Active, spontaneous speech is particularly difficult. The vocabulary is poor, and sound pronunciation is impaired for many reasons (underdevelopment of the upper jaw, macroglossia, dental pathology, etc.).

Emotions in patients with Down syndrome are poorly differentiated, children are not independent, do not show initiative, very suggestible, prone to imitation, impulsive, often show negativism (especially to everything new) and unmotivated stubbornness.

In general, however, the emotional sphere is more preserved than intelligence. Children with Down syndrome are good at distinguishing the attitudes of others, many are responsive and caring in their own way, and they are characterised by feelings of shame, resentment, embarrassment and empathy.

Different - both eretically and torpidly - can be temperament.

Eretic children are fidgety, restless, very curious and interfere in everything, sociable, but fearful of many things, especially novelty. In relations with others are often affectionate, willingly talk, can use gesture. Joyfully perceive praise, jealous, demand attention to themselves and do not like it to draw attention to others. At the same time, these children can be irritable and angry, able to sneak offence to the weak.

For the most part, though, they are still friendly and helpful.

Torpid children are sedentary, motor awkward, withdrawn, indifferent, when attempting to engage in conversation, they answer one-wordedly and often inappropriately ("I forgot", "I don't know", "I don't remember", etc.). They are slow to engage in work, but if they do, they work very diligently and are assiduous. Emotional features can be very different.

Life cycle dynamics are characteristic.

The period of maturation passes with great delay and total underdevelopment (children begin to fix their gaze at the age of about one year, hold their head - at about 8 months, sit - after a year, walk - at 2-3 years, etc.), the period of maturity is short (from 17-20 to 3040 years), after which signs of senile involution appear and rapidly increase.

Down syndrome has received a lot of attention not only because it is more common than other chromosomal disorders. Here we see an example of how knowledge of clinical features (tendency to imitation, curiosity, in some children - diligence, greater preservation of the emotional sphere, etc.) allows us to choose reference positions for the construction of the educational and correctional process, to predict the pupil's behaviour, taking into account possible manifestations of irritability, rudeness, increased sexuality, mood instability in the pubertal period, combined with some growth of intellectual potential.

When the number of sex chromosomes is disturbed, somatic and mental abnormalities are less severe than when the number of autosomes is disturbed. In these cases, mental retardation is often absent or manifested in mild forms; malformations, if any, are not severe; however, disorders of the emotional-volitional sphere are usually clearly delineated and often occupy an important (if not leading) place in the clinical picture.

An example of abnormalities in the sex chromosome system is ***Sherechevsky-Turner syndrome,*** or monosomy on the X chromosome

(45, XO).

Sensory pathology is quite common: 22% have visual impairment (myopia) and 52% have sensorineural hearing loss. Mental underdevelopment (mild, rarely moderate degree) is found in 16-25% of patients. Another part of patients with the Shereshevsky-Turner syndrome is characterised by a peculiar worldly practicalism, submissiveness, narrowness of interests, and low productivity of thinking.

In character, girls with Shereshevsky-Turner syndrome are complacent, hard-working, often inclined to teach and resonance, like to patronise the younger ones, to take care of the house. In puberty or prepubertal period often occur neurotic reactions associated with the realisation of their inferiority, with the experience of defect; girls become withdrawn, irritable, often rude.

Some of the undesirable manifestations can be prevented and corrected by timely estrogen treatment.

In general, mental retardation in combination with craniofacial dysmorphies and malformations of internal organs is characteristic of the clinical picture of most chromosomal diseases, including quantitative and structural abnormalities.

6.2. MENTAL RETARDATION IN MONOGENIC DISEASES

Monogenic diseases are a heterogeneous group of conditions that differ both in the specificity of mutations, peculiarities of pathogenesis, and clinical picture. The group of monogenic diseases with mental retardation includes some hereditary metabolic diseases, connective tissue diseases, isolated forms of microcephaly, hydrocephalus and a number of other diseases.

As noted above, hereditary metabolic defects, in particular enzymopathies or enzymopathies, constitute a large group of monogenically inherited diseases. By the beginning of XXI century more than 100 enzymopathies are known, and for more than 40 of them methods of drug therapy or dietary treatment have been developed in principle. Early diagnosis and timely treatment allow in most cases to prevent brain damage (and, consequently, intellectual underdevelopment) at those stages of its formation, when it is particularly vulnerable. Enzymopathies are inherited most often autosomal recessive or X-linked recessive, their frequency varies widely (from 1:1000 to 1:1 000000).

The central pathogenetic link of an enzymopathy is the absence or significant decrease in the activity of a particular enzyme, which blocks or causes a significant deficiency of a particular biochemical process. Since most enzyme systems are multicomponent, enzymopathies are usually represented by several genetic forms. It should also be considered that the enzyme is almost always involved in more than one metabolic pathway, making the disease polysymptomatic, affecting several organ systems. Accordingly, isolated intellectual impairment is rare; among other systems, vision is particularly frequently affected (in galactosemia, homocystinuria, mucopolysaccharidosis, amaurotic idiocy, etc.).

One of the most frequent (average 1:10000) and well-studied enzymopathies is ***phenylketonuria (PKU),*** phenylpyruvic oligophrenia, Fölling's disease). The main consequence of the toxic effect of phenylketo acids is mental retardation (in 65% - profound, in 31.8% - moderate and severe, and only in 3.2% - mild). Phenylpyruvic acid is excreted with urine, giving it a special "mouse" ("wolf") odour.

Tyrosine deficiency affects the formation of melanin pigment, while the metabolism of thyroid hormones and catecholamines is affected to a lesser extent. In this regard, patients with FCU have depigmented (or poorly pigmented) skin, increased sensitivity to ultraviolet light, often develop eczema and dermatitis; hair is light and iris colour is light. The skull (especially its cerebral part) is underdeveloped (secondary microcephaly). A specific posture is characteristic: elbow, hip and knee joints are slightly bent, the torso is tilted forward. Pathological anatomy reveals low brain mass, defects of myelination in the cerebral cortex (especially in the frontal and temporal lobes) and other structures (internal capsule, visual conductive pathways), depigmentation of the substantia nigra.

Psychopathological Apart from mental retardation, there is underdevelopment of speech (there is either no speech at all, or there are separate words that patients do not relate to objects), speech comprehension and pronunciation are sharply disturbed.

Neurological symptoms are nonspecific: epi- leptiform seizures, muscle tone disorders, poor coordination of movements, many stereotypies, other signs of extrapyramidal insufficiency (athetoid, choreiform movements) are frequent.

The behaviour of patients varies. In some cases, it is close to field behaviour (motor restlessness, untargeted, uncontrolled movements from object to object, aimless manipulation of objects, etc.). In other cases, children are passive, lethargic, do not show a sense of attachment, do not recognise loved ones well, and become animated mainly at the mention of food.

In untreated cases, the first manifestations are detected most often 2-3 months after birth (rarely earlier), and in general, the dynamics of the disease does not fit into purely evolutionary patterns.

Impaired intellectual development is also shown in some heterozygous carriers of the FKU gene. When the fact of heterozygous carriage was confirmed in parents and sibs of patients, mild intellectual disability was detected in 4% of cases, and in 6.5% - the lower limit of normal intelligence with a corresponding low level of education, professional and social adaptation.

The beginning of dietary treatment (exclusion of products containing phenylalanine) in the first weeks of life and its implementation for 10-12 years allows in about 90% of cases to prevent the development of mental retardation; if treatment is started at an older age, the development of intellectual disability can not be prevented, but behaviour is somewhat normalised, less frequent "epileptic seizures".

The successful use of medication and nutritional therapy in FCU is one of the most striking examples of medical correction and prevention of developmental abnormalities.

Another example of the same group of disorders is ***homocystinuria,*** in which the appearance of the patients resembles Marfan syndrome. The incidence of homocystinuria ranges from 1:50,000 to 1:250,000.

The minimum diagnostic features are a marfanoid phenotype, increased plasma concentrations of methionine and homocystine combined with a decrease in the same for cystine, and increased urinary excretion of homocystine (homocystinuria).

The pathogenesis of homocystinuria is based on a disorder in the metabolism of sulphur-containing amino acids. Normally, one of these amino acids, methionine, is converted to cysteine through a number of intermediate stages (including homo-cysteine and cystathionine).

Currently, 4 forms of homocystinuria are known, and in most cases there is a deficiency of the enzyme cystathionine beta-synthase, resulting in an increase in the content of homocystine (a derivative of homocysteine) and sometimes methionine in the blood, tissues and urine. Increased concentration of these substances natural to the body causes focal necrosis in the kidneys, spleen, gastric mucosa, blood vessels. Damage to vessel walls, as well as activation of the blood coagulation system increases thrombosis, which is manifested by thrombosis of coronary, carotid, renal arteries, generalised venous thrombosis. This can lead to arterial hypertension, various neurological disorders, early death.

Homocystinuria is also characterised by elongation of tubular bones, funnel-shaped or keel-shaped chest deformity, scoliosis, kyphosis, valgus deformity of knee joints and/or feet, flat feet, changes in the shape and location of teeth, as well as osteoporosis, tendency to fractures, and limitation of joint mobility. Some patients have lens subluxation, sometimes accompanied by myopia, optic atrophy, retinal detachment and glaucoma.

Neurologically, various signs of focal pathology (hemiparesis, hemiplegia, less often seizure) and gait disorders are detected. These disorders often have a progressive character. There is also a poor switchability of attention, reduced efficiency, uncriticalness of self and others. Speech is a limited set of short agrammatical phrases, sound pronunciation disorders are common, reduced vocabulary. The vast majority of patients have reduced intelligence (1Q from 70 to 30, i.e. from mild to severe intellectual deficiency).

Similar, although more polymorphic, clinical manifestations are characteristic of other forms of homocystinuria caused by disorders of the coenzyme systems of metabolism of sulfur-containing amino acids. The disease is inherited autosomal recessively. The homocystinuria gene is localised in the long arm of chromosome 21.

In some diseases (they are called "accumulation diseases") the enzymes of catabolism of some substances are affected, as a result of which the latter accumulate in cells, disrupting all their vital activity. Examples are mucopolysaccharidoses, Niemann-Pick disease, etc.

For example, in ***Niemann-Pick disease*** (inherited autosomal recessively, occurs equally often in boys and girls), there is a deficiency of acid sphingomyelinidase and the metabolism of one type of lipid, sphingomyelin, is disturbed. Products of its incomplete breakdown accumulate in the cells of the liver, spleen, brain, lymph nodes, lymphocytes. There are several forms of the disease, differing clinically (in time of onset, severity of visceral and neuropsychiatric manifestations), and, apparently, non-identical genetically. Common symptoms are enlargement of the liver and spleen, and generalised enlargement of lymph nodes. At the early onset of the disease visceral signs rapidly increase, mental and physical development is grossly delayed, neurological disorders rapidly progress, and patients die at the age of 3-5 years. In the juvenile form, in addition to visceral symptoms, there are signs of nervous system damage (seizures, cerebellar symptoms, etc.), but they appear late, develop slowly. In the visceral form, the nervous system is not affected.

Monogenic forms of oligophrenia include ***true microcephaly and obturator hydrocephalus.***

Small brain size is found in at least 2.5 per cent of children with intellectual disability. The causes of microcephaly may vary; $1/_{10}$ part of such cases are not associated with exogenous lesions of the intrauterine period and belong to genetically determined "true" microcephaly, which is inherited autosomal recessively. These patients usually have profound general mental underdevelopment, and often also seizures and cerebral motor disorders.

The recessive gene for true microcephaly is present in about 10% of heterozygous carriers, and its features include reduced skull size and mild intellectual deficits. Some experts believe that up to 10% of all cases of clinically identified intellectual disability are due to heterozygosity for the true microcephaly gene.

Hereditary obturator hydrocephalus accounts for approximately *1/3 of* all cases of congenital hydrocephalus. Inheritance is more often X-linked recessive (i.e. occurs only in boys), but autosomal dominant and autosomal recessive inheritance are known. Regardless of the type of inheritance, the main pathogenetic point is stenosis of the sylvian aqueduct. The absence of normal conditions for cerebrospinal fluid outflow from the first three cerebral ventricles causes trogredient neurological symptoms, and without surgical repair of the defect at an early age, the prognosis is unfavourable.

Martin-Bell syndrome (X-chromosome breakage syndrome) is a hereditary disease with mental retardation. The syndrome is inherited X-linked recessively and occurs mainly in boys, although it is also found in *1/3 of* female carriers of the gene. Its frequency is 1:1250- 1:5000 males. At present, the nature of genetic changes underlying this disease has been elucidated. It has been shown that the clinical manifestations of the syndrome are associated with an increase in the number of trinucleotide repeats of cytosine-guanine-guanine on a certain section of the long arm of the X chromosome (Xq27.3).

Example. The first child in the family, a boy (at the time of the examination at the age of 18), suffers from Martin-Bell syndrome. His intellect corresponds to a pronounced mental retardation, autism is noted;

despite officially recognised learning disability, in the conditions of a special institution for children with autism he managed to form speech, writing, reading and everyday skills; being musical, the child has mastered elementary skills of playing the piano. During the year he worked as a caretaker and office cleaner; he coped with the work satisfactorily, but required constant supervision. His level of social adaptation excluded the possibility of independent living.

The parents sought medical and genetic counselling due to the desire to have a second child. The probability of having a Free child and measures to control the course of the pregnancy were determined. Investigations during the subsequent pregnancy (male foetus) were positive for the presence of X-chromosome breakage syndrome, and the pregnancy was terminated; pathomorphological studies fully confirmed the correctness of the prenatal diagnosis.

A third pregnancy, also under medical genetic monitoring, resulted in the birth of a normal girl, and a five-year follow-up indicates that the child has no significant mental or physical developmental deficits.

Among the diverse forms of mental retardation of monogenic nature are the so-called xerodermic forms, in which the intellectual defect is combined with skin lesions. Examples of these diseases are neurofibromatosis and tuberous sclerosis.

Neurofibromatosis ***(Recklinghausep's disease)*** is characterised by multiple tumours along the course of peripheral nerves, tumours of the central nervous system, visual organs, internal organs, skin pigmentation, cutaneous nevi, and bone anomalies.

The unfolded form of neurofibromatosis occurs at an incidence of 1:2500-1:3000 neonates, is inherited autosomal dominantly with 100% penetrance and variable expressivity.

Two forms of neurofibromatosis are currently distinguished; the classic peripheral form (neurofibromatosis I), the gene for which is localised on chromosome 17, and the central form (neurofibromatosis II), the gene for which is located on chromosome 22.

Minimum diagnostic signs of neurofibromatosis: presence of more than 5 "coffee and milk coloured" spots on the skin with a diameter of at least 15 mm; two or more neurofibromas; optic nerve glioma.

The disease is manifested from birth or in the first decade of life by pigment spots on the skin, which gradually increase in size and number (Fig. 45a). The spots are most often localised on closed areas of the skin (on the back and sides of the trunk, as well as in the axillary and inguinal areas). Cutaneous and subcutaneous tumours are located along the course of peripheral nerves (Fig. 456). Gliomas of the optic nerve are most characteristic, and neurofibromas may occur on the eyelids, conjunctiva, cornea, and iris. If tumours arise inside the orbits, they can provoke ptosis, paralysis of eye muscles. Skeletal disorders (kyphosis, scoliosis, tubular bone disorders, etc.) are less common.

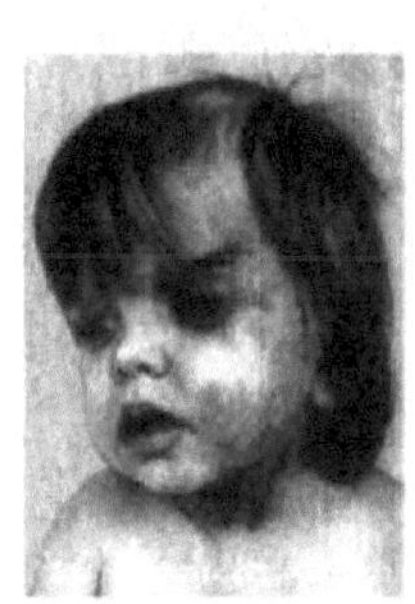

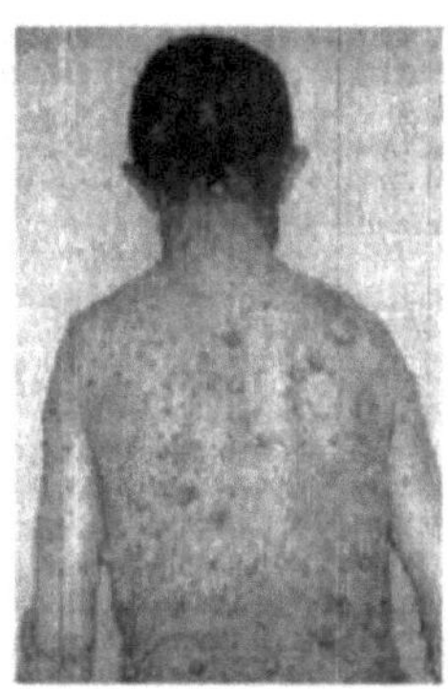

aah

Fig.45. Recklinghausen's neurofibrimotosis: a- pigment spots on the skin of a child; b- skin tumours in an adult patient.

Lesions of the nervous system are diverse in spectrum, severity and dynamics, which is determined by the localisation and size of neoplasms. One of the manifestations of their localisation in the central nervous system is a decrease in intelligence, impaired memory, attention, sometimes convulsive syndrome. These signs may not be manifested in all patients, they begin with minor manifestations, but, gradually increasing, lead to speech disorders, weakening of some higher mental functions and, as a consequence, to difficulties in learning. Over time, in many cases, school problems increase, are aggravated by personality deviations, and may lead to transfer to lower-level programmes (and, accordingly, to a special (remedial) school of the VIII type) and/or individual education.

A characteristic feature of neurofibromatosis type II is the formation of tumours of the cranial nerves and spinal cord.

The clinical picture is dominated by various neurological disorders, progressive decline in intelligence and mental disintegration in general. Cutaneous tumours and peripheral neurofibromas are usually absent. For special pedagogy, this type of disease has no significant significance.

The minimum diagnostic features of ***tuberous sclerosis (Burneyville-***

Pringle disease) are facial angiofibroma, seizures and mental retardation (Figure 46). The incidence of tuberous sclerosis at birth is approximately 1:10,000, in the general population it ranges from 1:30,000 to 1:100,000. 80% of cases are associated with a mutation; the mechanism of inheritance is autosomal dominant with 100% penetrance and variable expression. The disease manifests at the age of 2-5 years most often (93%) with seizures of various types (grand mal, petit mal, Salaam, etc.). Of other neurological disorders are hydrocephalus, pyramidal and extrapyramidal symptoms. In the brain - in the walls of the ventricles, cerebellum, basal ganglia numerous calcifications are found.

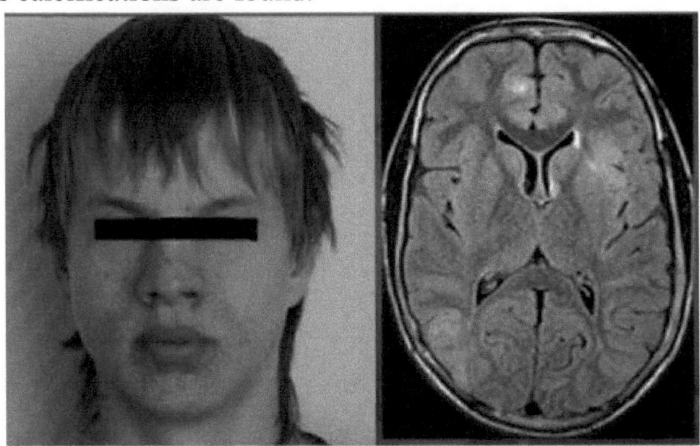

Figure 46. Tuberous sclerosis. Butterfly-shaped skin lesions on the cheeks, shagreen thickening of the skin, pigmented and depigmented irregularly shaped spots.

Mental retardation is found in about /$^{3}_{4}$ cases and can vary from mild to severe. Its structure also varies: in one part of cases, underdevelopmental phenomena prevail with the preservation of the hierarchical structure typical of an oligophrenic defect, while in another part, the procedural 156 dementia. In terms of skin lesions, these are primarily (70% of cases) angiofibroma of the cheeks in the form of "butterfly" (red and pink papules), shagreen skin, depigmented spots, coffee spots, subcutaneous fibromatous nodules, etc. In the visual system there are tumour-like changes of the retina, sometimes glaucoma.

Both benign and malignant tumours of various organs are significantly more common than the population average. The course of the disease is progressive, and most patients die at 20-25 years of age.

6.3. MULTIFACTORIAL MENTAL RETARDATION

This type of mental retardation is currently poorly understood. It is believed to be inherited on the basis of additive (summative) action of many genes (hereditary component or predisposition) and environmental factors (non-hereditary component), which prevents normal intellectual development of the child. This form seems to be common. As a rule, there are no neurological disorders, no obvious morphological abnormalities, and intellectual disability is almost always mild in degree and uncomplicated in structure.

Thus, hereditary mental retardation is diverse in its clinical manifestations and genetic nature. Exogenous factors are three times less likely than genetic factors to be the direct cause of intellectual developmental disorders, but they can become a condition for the manifestation of genetic pathology.

6.4. MENTAL RETARDATION

Mental retardation (MRD) is a clinically polymorphic form of developmental abnormalities, the main feature of which is immaturity of the emotional-volitional sphere and cognitive activity: the main characteristics of mental activity of children with MRD of a certain age are close to the characteristics typical of children of an earlier, previous age stage of development.

The aetiology of ZPD is heterogeneous. The differences in the etiopathogenesis of ZPD are the basis for the most widespread 157 currently used classification. According to this classification, constitutional, somatogenic, psychogenic and residual-organic forms of ZPD are distinguished.

There are practically no works specifically devoted to the role of genetic factors in the aetiology of ZPD, and this is not surprising: the symptoms observed in this developmental abnormality are not of a severe, gross nature, occur in a wide variety of spectrum and degree of severity of combinations and relate mainly to higher mental functions, the mechanisms of transmission of which from generation to generation are not sufficiently studied.

Genetic factors are undoubtedly significant in the case of constitutional forms of ZPD. This is confirmed by the repetition in a number of generations of the features of physique and personality traits characteristic (including those typical of ZPD).

The role of hereditary factors in somatogenic ZPD is most often determined by the underlying somatic disease.
Genetic factors play the greatest role in the aetiology of ZPD of residual-organic genesis.

6.5. EARLY INFANTILE AUTISM

In ***early childhood autism (ECA),*** the child's ability to interact with the world around him or her, and above all with other people, is impaired. Forced self-isolation leads to impaired development of the emotional sphere, speech, cognitive functions, and the psyche as a whole. Childhood autism occurs quite often, 20-25 cases per 10000 newborns (including mild forms, according to recent data, up to 40-45 per 10000), with boys 4-4.5 times more often than girls. Approximately 70% of autistic children have mental retardation with 10 less than 70 and 30% with 10 less than 50. Despite the high incidence of mental retardation among children with autism, the type of cognitive defect in autism differs from mental retardation in non-autistic individuals.
The first signs of autism may appear as early as infancy in the form of a lack of an animation complex when in contact with the mother and other loved ones. At an older age, autism manifests *itself in "withdrawal into itself",* in a decrease or complete absence of contact with the outside world. The child does not participate in conversation, does not answer questions. Weakness and poverty of emotional reactions are characteristic. Along with this, for patients 158
Autism is characterised by hypersensitivity to light, sound and other stimuli, and a constant sense of fear. There is a tendency to stereotyped movements and motor deficiencies.
The etiology of RDA is not clear enough, but it is obvious that it is heterogeneous. It is shown that organic brain lesions play a certain role, but it is difficult to speak about the localisation of disorders at present. The most frequently detected are disorders of cortical-subcortical connections, mediobasal sections of the frontal lobes, interhemispheric interaction, hypoplasia of some parts of the cerebellar worm. The role of these symptoms in the pathogenesis of autism remains unclear, and it is generally difficult to judge whether organic disorders are a manifest factor or a complicating syndrome in some cases of autism.
At the same time, it should be noted that in the last 10-15 years, according to the observations of both foreign and domestic clinicians, the frequency and severity of signs of organic brain damage in autism is increasing.

It is possible that psychogenic factors also play a role, but, apparently, they are only one of the possible manifest influences, or they form neurotic layering both in autism itself and in secondary autism in children with other developmental disorders - sensory disorders, infantile cerebral palsy, some speech disorders (alalia, open rhinolalia, severe forms of stuttering), less often in ZPD.

The role of genetic factors is widely recognised, and virtually all prominent researchers on the biological basis of autism now agree that a significant proportion of ADA cases (if not all) are hereditary. This is indicated by a number of observations.

Childhood autism is often combined with chromosomal diseases: cases of autism with chromosome number abnormalities have been described, and the combination of AD with gene diseases (phenylketonuria, tuberous sclerosis, neurofibromatosis, etc.) is quite common. A special role is attributed to the X-chromosome breakage syndrome: according to some researchers, on average, one out of 4-5 boys with autism suffers from the X-chromosome breakage syndrome (see above).

The role of genetic factors in the development of autism is also indicated by the results of twin studies. According to these findings, there are significant differences in concordance in autism 159
(the probability of a disease or trait occurring in one member of a twin pair given the presence of that disease or trait in the other member) for monozygotic (genetically identical) and dizygotic (genetically dissimilar) twin pairs. For monozygotic twins, *the* concordance rate is 90-93%, whereas for dizygotic twins it is 0-10%, indicating a very large role of the hereditary factor. At the same time, the concordance in monozygotic twins does not reach 100%, which is considered as an indication of a certain role of exogenous factors and, possibly, the polytene nature of inheritance. It is important to note that the study was not conducted on the population of special schools for autistic children, but included all twins in Sweden, Norway, Denmark, Finland and Iceland.

The mechanism of inheritance of the disease is unclear, but it is obviously not monogenic: numerous attempts to "fit" practical observations into the scheme of autosomal recessive, X-linked recessive inheritance have not been successful. A multifactorial mechanism is considered to be the most probable (i.e. the gene complex provides transmission of predisposition to the development of pathology, but it is realised only in the presence of a non-specific exogenous or endogenous factor). This point of view is attractive because it is the best way to explain the temporal and/or substantive relationship with a variety of exogenous factors and the exceptionally large clinical polymorphism of the RDA syndrome. The latter is especially interesting if we accept V.P. Efroimson's hypothesis that the clinical manifestation of a polygenic complex can be caused by the presence of at least one pathological gene, i.e. it is not necessarily the presence of the whole complex or a certain part of it. The same hypothesis helps to explain the growth of the number of patients with autism, despite the fact that the patients themselves do not leave offspring.

The subtle genetic mechanisms of RDA inheritance are poorly understood. Some studies have convincingly demonstrated the association of artistic disorders with the c-Harvey-ra8 (HRAS) gene localised in the short arm of chromosome 11 (11p15.5), or, more precisely, with the frequency of its BZ/BZ allele ratio. The authors draw attention to the role of ras-protein in the processes of growth of neural structures, mechanisms of nerve transmission, intracellular transport and cytoarchitectonics of the central nervous system.

A series of other papers draw attention to a possible link between autism and microduplication of the GABRB3 gene, localised in the short arm of the 15th chromosome (15p+) and apparently acting through changes in the structure of the serotonin transport protein.

Thus, both groups of works allow us to identify guanine triphosphate-dependent systems, nerve growth factor, cholinergic systems, and the sympathetic system as potential links in the pathogenesis of RDA, although, unfortunately, it is currently impossible to give a more complete and accurate characterisation of the place and importance of these systems in the pathogenesis of RDA. At the same time, the means of pharmacological influence on these systems (primarily on the sympathetic system and cholinergic structures) are well known, and their use in clinical practice can be attributed to pathogenetic means of treatment with some caution.

Moreover, careful analysis of the effects of agents acting on certain links in the pathogenetic chain may, in principle, provide new information about the pathogenesis of autism itself.

6.6. PERMANENT HEARING LOSS

Persistent hearing loss includes ***deafness and hearing loss***.

In ***deafness***, due to a disorder of the neurosensory systems (the cortical organ and/or the nervous apparatus of the auditory analyser), the perception of audible speech by ear alone is impossible under any circumstances, since not only the threshold of auditory perception is significantly raised, but also the frequency range of perceived sounds is limited (to 3.5-4 kHz or less). Depending on the severity of the lesion, some non-speech sounds, individual phonemes, familiar words and even phrases may be perceived in such disorders, but speech in general is inaccessible. Total deafness (when no sounds are perceived) accounts for no more than 2-3% of all cases of this pathology.

In hearing loss, speech perception is difficult, but under special conditions (sound amplification) is possible, because the shortening of the tone scale does not affect the speech frequency range, although the threshold of auditory perception is raised by 30-80 dB.

It should be noted that while in medicine they sometimes speak of "temporary deafness" or "temporary hearing loss", in special (correctional) pedagogy they mean not transient, but persistent, inaccessible to medical treatment. If they develop in childhood, it inevitably has a negative impact on speech development, on the formation of personality and psyche as a whole. A condition arises that includes not only hearing impairment, but also numerous neurological and psychopathological symptoms (many of which can be corrected with timely and adequate work).

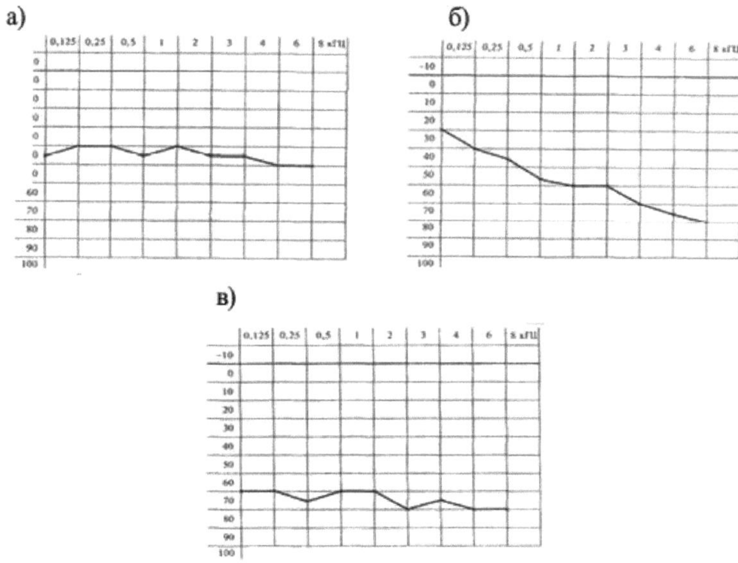

Graph-1. ***Hearing Losses (dB).***

(a) Typical audiogram for monogenic autosomal recessive hearing loss.

b) Typical audiogram for monogenic autosomal dominant hearing loss.
c) Typical audiogram for monogenic X-linked recessive hearing loss.
According to the data of domestic authors, about 60% of all isolated hearing impairments are caused by genetic factors. Inheritance is most often monogenic, with autosomal recessive type being inherited in about 80% of cases of sensorineural hearing impairment, 19% - in autosomal dominant type and 1% - in X-linked recessive type. With significant polymorphism of the audiometric picture in the first of the mentioned cases, a uniform increase in the threshold of auditory perception by 45-50 dB (*a*) within the entire speech frequency range is typical, in the second case the audiogram has a descending character (in the low-frequency part of the speech range the hearing threshold is raised by 30-35 dB *(b),* in the high-frequency area (3-5 kHz) - up to 80 and more dB) and in the third case - a uniform decrease to 70-80 and more dB (*c*) throughout the entire tonescale is typical (Diagram-1. *Hearing reductions, (dB)).*
Many clinically similar persistent hearing disorders are genetically heterogeneous. For example, otosclerosis, which is characterised by progressive hearing loss developing at a young age due to limitation of stapes mobility, accompanied by tinnitus and sometimes dizziness, is inherited in most cases by autosomal dominant type with incomplete penetrance, but other types of inheritance have also been described.
The numerous syndromal forms of persistent hearing impairment are classified by B.V. Konigsmark and R.D. Gordin according to the main concomitant feature. They identified 8 main groups in which persistent hearing impairment is combined with other defects, such as:

Examples of microtia

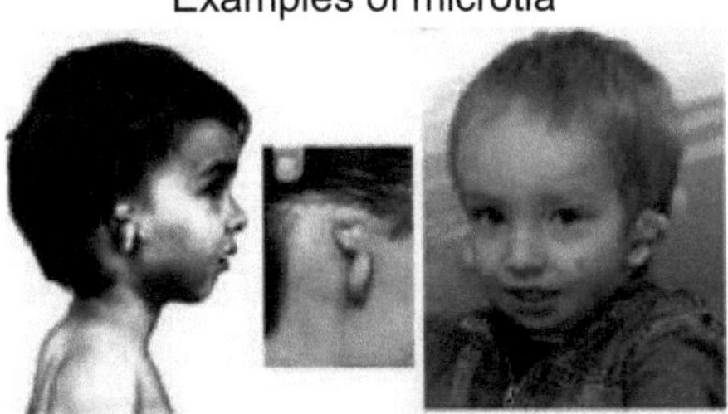

Figure 47. Microtia syndrome with atresia of the external auditory canal and conductive deafness. Severe deformity of the auricle.

1) anomalies of the external ear. One example of this group of disorders is ***microtia with atresia of the external auditory canal and conductive hearing loss*** (Fig. 47). The disease is manifested by various deformities or

absence of the auricle; atresia of the external auditory canal is sometimes found; hearing loss is more often conductive, rarely neurosensory; the type of inheritance is presumably autosomal recessive;

2) malformations and diseases of the visual organs. An example is ***Usher syndrome, which*** occurs in 2.5 per cent of deaf people (congenital sensorineural deafness and retinitis pigmentosa). Congenital sensorineural hearing loss, lack of vestibular responses, and slowly progressive retinitis pigmentosa with onset in the 1st or 2nd decade of life are typical. Other ocular symptoms include cataracts, retinal degeneration, and sometimes glaucoma. In a quarter of cases - mental retardation, sometimes schizophrenia. It is inherited autosomal recessively;

3) skeletal malformations and connective tissue diseases. Among this group of persistent hearing impairments, two characteristic diseases can be distinguished: craniofacial dysostosis, or ***Crouzon syndrome***, and mandibular-facial dysostosis, or ***Treacher-Collins syndrome.***

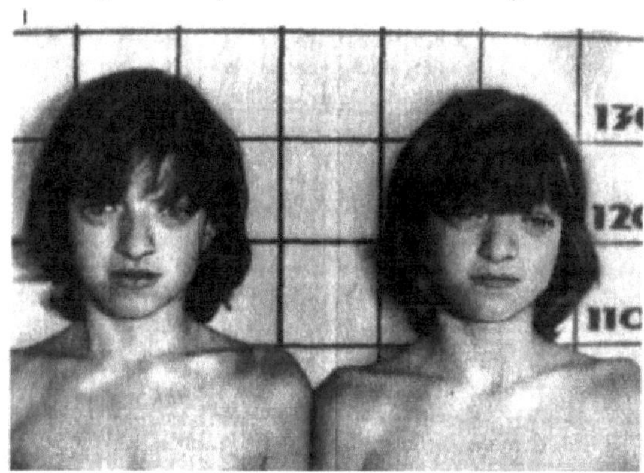

Figure 48. Craniofacial dysostosis of Croozon. Hypertelorism, exophthalmos, divergent strabismus, hypoplasia of the maxilla.

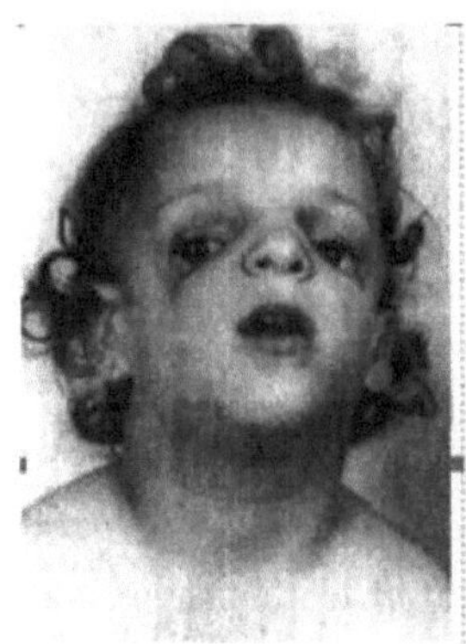

Figure 49. Titcher-Collins syndrome. Antimongoloid eyes, hypoplasia of zygomatic bones and orbits, anomaly of ears.

The main manifestations of Crouzon syndrome are skull deformities (brachycephaly, oxycephaly), exophthalmos, small orbits, hypoplasia of the maxilla (Fig. 48). Hypertelorism, divergent strabismus, nystagmus, beak-like nose, sometimes cleft palate or uvula, bilateral atresia of the external auditory canal, and various degrees of hearing, intellectual, and visual impairment are also observed. The type of inheritance is autosomal dominant.

The main clinical manifestations of ***Treacher-Collins syndrome*** are bilateral hypoplasia of the zygomatic bones and orbits, coloboma of the lower eyelids, antimongoloid cut of the eye slits, absence of eyelashes on the lower eyelid, anomalies of the auricles, conductive deafness, and hypoplasia of the mandible (Fig. 49). The type of inheritance is autosomal dominant;

4) abnormal kidney function. An example is ***hereditary nephritis with deafness, or Alport syndrome.*** The disease is manifested by various renal dysfunctions (haematuria, proteinuria, etc.), often progressing to renal failure. In 50% of cases there are neurosensory hearing disorders, beginning from the first years of life. In 15% of patients cataract or other diseases are detected.

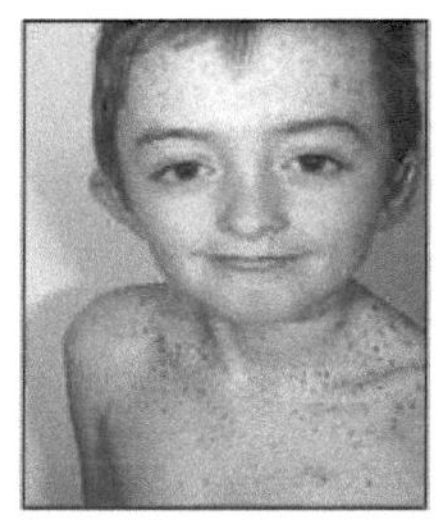

Eye anomalies. Genetic heterogeneity of the syndrome is assumed (6 forms with different clinical features and different types of inheritance - autosomal dominant, X-linked recessive, autosomal recessive).
Alport syndrome occurs in 1% of children with congenital hearing loss;
5) endocrine pathology. This group of diseases includes the persistent combination of goitre with sensorineural deafness. The disease is called ***Pendred syndrome***, which occurs in 10% of patients with congenital deafness. The disease is characterised by congenital sensorineural deafness. From the age of 5-8 years, there is an increase in the thyroid gland due to the development of diffuse goitre. In some cases, mental retardation is observed. It is inherited autosomal recessively;
6) pathology of the nervous system, such as ataxia, hypogonadism, mental retardation and sensorineural deafness, called ***Richards-Rundle syndrome.*** Patients are characterised by delayed motor development, ataxia, underdevelopment of secondary sexual characteristics, foot deformities, claw-like deformity of the hand, kyphoscoliosis, muscle atrophy, mental retardation. Deafness is progressive in nature. The type of inheritance of the syndrome is autosomal recessive;
7) pathology of the cardiovascular system. In 1.5% of children with congenital deafness, ***Gervell and Lange-Nielsen syndrome*** is detected.

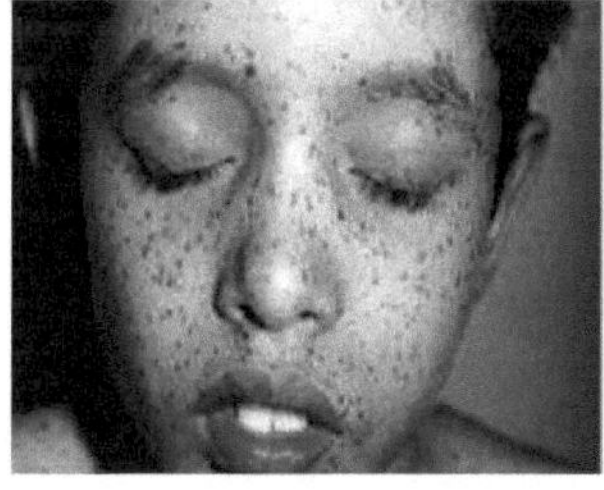

The syndrome is characterised by bilateral sensorineural deafness, attacks of loss of consciousness associated with physical exertion or nervous overexcitement. The ECG shows signs of cardiac conduction disturbances. More than half of patients die before the age of 14 years with cardiac arrhythmia.

Figure 50. Multiple lentigo syndrome.

Multiple small, flat, hyperpigmented hyperpigmented elements on the skin.

It's inherited autosomal recessively.

8) skin lesions and pigmentation disorders. An example of the combination of sensorineural deafness and skin lesions is the ***multiple lentigo syndrome*** (Fig. 50). In addition to these features, patients have growth retardation, hypertelorism, genital anomalies (cryptorchidism, hypospadias, hypogonadism), and pulmonary artery stenosis. The type of inheritance is auto-somnodominant with high penetrance. Another example is ***Waardenburg syndrome, with*** an incidence of a case per 4000 newborns. Typical manifestations of the syndrome include partial albinism, white strand of hair, telecanthus, wide protruding bridge of the nose, fused eyebrows, iris heterochrony, and patches of depigmentation on the skin (Fig. 51-A). Hypoplasia of the cortical organ results in sensorineural deafness or severe hearing loss. Waardenburg syndrome is inherited autosomal dominant with incomplete penetrance.

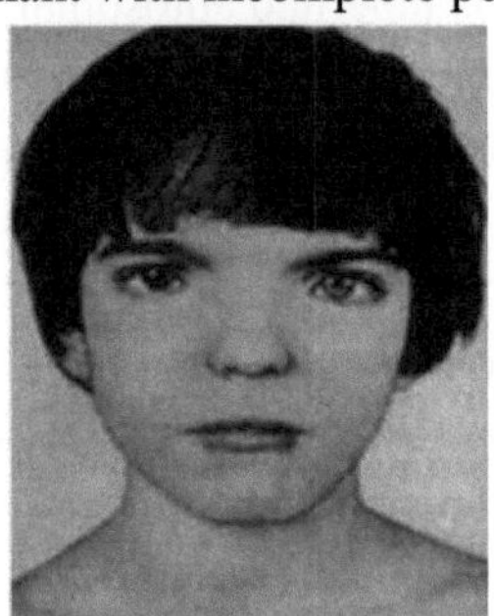

Figure 51-A. Waardenburg syndrome.

Telecanthus, wide nose bridge, iris heterochromia, white strand of hair.

6.7. PERMANENT VISUAL IMPAIRMENT

Persistent visual impairment includes ***blindness and low vision.***

Blind (blind) are persons with visual impairments in which visual sensations are either completely absent or there is light perception or residual vision (up to 0.04 in the better seeing eye with correction by glasses), as well as persons with progressive diseases and narrowing of the visual field (up to 10-15%) with visual acuity up to 0.08.

In low vision, visual acuity in the better seeing eye is between 0.5 and 0.2, corrected with ordinary glasses. In addition to reduced visual acuity,

visually impaired persons may have colour perception, peripheral vision and binocular vision.
Early development of blindness or low vision causes deviations in the motor sphere, in neuropsychological development. Many of these deviations can be corrected quite well.
According to domestic authors, 84.5 per cent of students in schools for blind and visually impaired children have congenital and, more often, hereditary disorders. It is believed that genetically determined visual impairments account for 60 to 80 per cent of all cases of this pathology, with autosomal recessive forms accounting for 80-90 per cent of cases.
Often persistent ophthalmological pathology is a component of hereditary syndromes (about 16% of cases of hereditary blindness and low vision). For example, various visual impairments and eye anomalies are found in ***Rieger syndrome.***

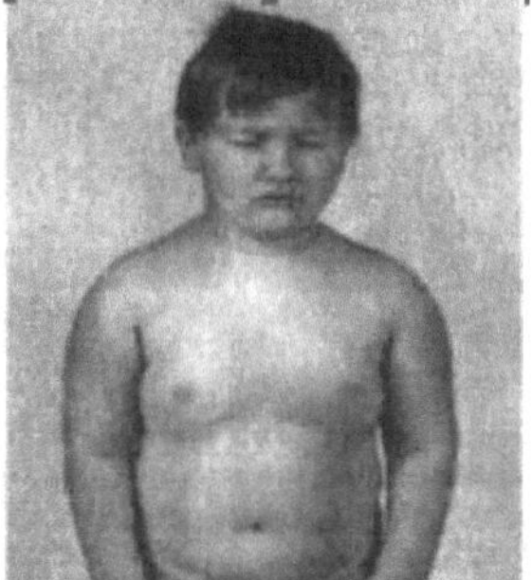

Figure 51-B. Alströn's syndrome.
Short stature, obesity, scrotal hypoplasia, eyes closed due to photophobia

The main manifestations of the syndrome are blueness of the sclera, aniridia, glaucoma, micro- or megalocornea, various iris disorders, corneal opacity, cataract, strabismus. There is a wide bridge of the nose, wide set eyes, turned lower lip, deformity of the auricles. The conical shape of the anterior teeth and oligodontia are also characteristic. The type of inheritance is autosomnodominant.
In ***Alströn syndrome***, nystagmus appears in the first year of life, and retinal inflammation and photophobia develop. There is a progressive decline in central and peripheral vision, leading to blindness by about 7 years of age. Patients are characterised by progressive hearing loss. Obesity is noted from early childhood (Fig. 51-B).
After puberty, there are signs of insulin-independent diabetes mellitus and

nephropathy leading to renal failure. Sexual development is outwardly normal, but testicular biopsy reveals aplasia of germinative cells and sclerosis of the seminal tubules. Intelligence is usually preserved. The type of inheritance is autosomal recessive.

The leading clinical manifestation of ***Lenz syndrome*** is usually unilateral microphthalmia or anophthalmia (Fig. 52). In addition, hand anomalies (syndactyly, doubling of the thumbs, etc.), moderate microcephaly, deformed, protruding, low-set auricles are characteristic. Patients

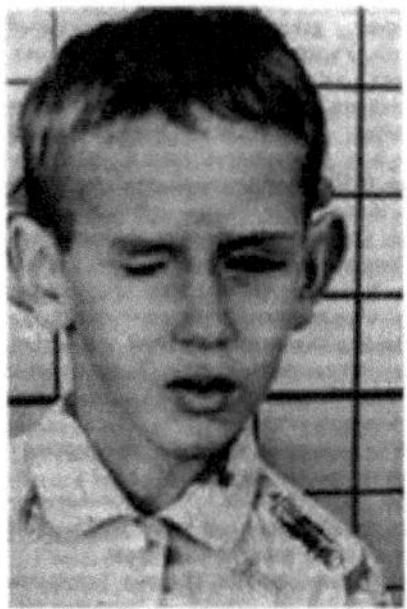

Figure 52. Lenz syndrome. Anophthalmia with protruding auricles.

Asthenic physique, with narrow shoulders and hips. Heart, gastrointestinal and renal malformations are common.

Bite disorders and partial adontia are also noted. Mental retardation is insignificant. Lenz syndrome is X-linked recessively inherited. Heterozygous carriers may have mild manifestations of the disease (hand anomalies, narrow face, dental anomalies, etc.).

Congenital cataracts are united on the basis of the leading feature - clouding of the lens. The clinical picture depends on

the intensity and localisation of opacity in the lens. About 25 per cent

in congenital cataracts is a complete nuclear cataract, which leads to a decrease in visual acuity, sometimes significantly. Layer cataract often leads to visual disability.

It accounts for up to 40% of all cases, usually affects both eyes, and develops with slow progression. Congenital cataracts with vision loss are accompanied by strabismus and nystagmus in 30% of cases. In 25% of cases unilateral and in 11% of cases bilateral cataracts are combined with microphthalmos. Congenital cataracts are inherited autosomal dominant, autosomal recessive, X-linked recessive. Visual impairment is also observed in the above-described Usher, Alythort, Marfan, Crouzon and many other syndromes, as well as in various hereditary metabolic disorders.

Control Questions and Assignments:

1. Which pathology is called hereditary?
2. Into which groups can all hereditary diseases be divided?
3. Give a brief characterisation of gene-based diseases?
4. How do genetic diseases arise?
5. What type of amino acid metabolism disease is inherited?
6. Give a brief characterisation of the clinical manifestations of amino acid metabolism disease?

TEST-6.

1. Which sex is called homogametic (a), which is called heterogametic (b). 1 - having two X chromosomes; 2 - having X and U chromosomes; 3 - in humans it is male; 4 - in chickens it is male.

a)a-1,4 6-2,3. b) a-1,3 6-2,4. c) a-2,3 6-1,4. e) a-2,46-1,3.

2. The marriage of a healthy man and a healthy woman gave birth to 6 sons: two with haemophilia, three with colour blindness, one with both haemophilia and colour blindness. Identify the genotype of the father.

a) XU, both genes are recessive in the X chromosome;

б) XU, in the X chromosome both genes are dominant;

в) XU, in the X chromosome the dominant gene for normal vision, in the U chromosome the dominant gene for normal coagulation;

e) XU, there is a recessive gene for normal vision in the X chromosome and a recessive gene for normal coagulation in the U chromosome.

3. Explain why the haemophilia gene always appears in males but is rarely seen in females?

a) the gene is recessive and located on the X chromosome;

б) the gene is dominant and located on the X chromosome;

в) the gene is recessive and located in the U chromosome;

e) the gene is dominant and located in the autosome.

4. Hypertrichosis is determined by a gene lying on the U chromosome, while one form of ichthyosis is recessive and linked to the X chromosome. In a family where the male has hypertrichosis and the female is healthy, a child with ichthyosis is born. Determine the probability of giving birth to sons without anomalies (in %).

(a) 75. 6)25. c) 50. e) 0.

5. A woman with normal teeth colour (a) and a man with dark teeth (A) have 4 daughters with dark teeth and 3 sons with white teeth. Determine

the pattern of inheritance of the trait.

a) the gene is located in the autosome; b) the gene is linked to the U chromosome;

c) the gene is X-linked; e) the gene is not fully dominant.

CHALLENGE-6.

1. Enamel hypoplasia is inherited as an X-linked dominant trait. In a family where both parents had this anomaly, a son was born with normal teeth.

What will their second son and daughter be like?

2. In humans, the gene that causes one of the forms of colour blindness or colour blindness is localised in the X chromosome. The disease state is caused by a recessive gene, the health state by a dominant gene. A girl with normal vision whose father had colour blindness marries a normal man whose father also had colour blindness.

What kind of vision can the children of this marriage have?

3. In humans, classical haemophilia is inherited as an X-linked recessive trait. Albinism is caused by an autosomal recessive gene. One couple normal for these two traits had a son with both abnormalities.

What is the probability that the second son in this family will also show both anomalies at the same time?

4. Make a symbolic record of the karyotypes of the following individuals:

1) a girl with Patau syndrome;
2) a boy with Edwards syndrome;
3) a boy with Down syndrome;
4) a boy with Klinefelter's syndrome;
5) a girl with shereshevsky-turner syndrome.

5. Transcribe the following karyotype records of diseased individuals:

1) 46, XX,lp+;
2) 46, Xy,14q-;
3) 46, XX,14p+;
4) 46, XX,del(l)(q21);
5) 45, Xy,t(14 q: 21q);
6) 46, XX,r(18).

CHAPTER VII

RESEARCH METHODS IN HUMAN GENETICS

To date, about 4,500 hereditary human diseases have been registered, and most of them are associated with mental disorders. According to the World Health Organisation (WHO), thanks to the use of new diagnostic methods, an average of three new hereditary diseases are registered annually, which are encountered in the practice of a doctor of any specialty: therapist, surgeon, neurologist, obstetrician-gynecologist, endocrinologist, etc.

Even within each speciality, hereditary diseases are numerous and diverse: there are over 300 hereditary diseases in neurology, over 250 in dermatology, and over 250 in ophthalmology. In addition, most forms of hereditary diseases are extremely rare (1 per 100,000 or less), and the doctor and nurse in their practice little or no such patients. It is not possible for a physician to have all the knowledge necessary to diagnose rare hereditary diseases, even within his speciality. Consequently, he must know the general principles of diagnosing hereditary diseases. These will enable him to suspect a hereditary disease in a patient and to carry out a "targeted" examination. Diseases that have absolutely nothing to do with heredity, virtually do not exist. The course of various diseases (viral, bacterial, mycoses and even traumas) and recovery from them depends to a greater or lesser extent on hereditary immunological, physiological, behavioural and mental characteristics of a person.

The task of medical genetics is the detection and prevention of hereditary diseases. The study of human heredity and variability is associated with difficulties, the main reasons for which are:

1) impossibility of directional crosses for subsequent genetic analyses;
2) the impossibility of experimentally obtaining mutations;
3) late puberty;
4) the small number of offspring in each family;
5) slow generational change;
6) the impossibility of providing the same and strictly controlled conditions for the development of offspring from different marriages;
7) insufficient accuracy of registration of hereditary traits and small pedigree;
8) complex karyotype (2p = 46) with a large number of linkage groups.

Despite all these difficulties, the progress in the knowledge of human

genetics in recent years is very great. The following methods are used in the study of heredity and variability in humans: genealogical, twin, population-static,
dermatoglyphic, biochemical, cytogenetic, somatic cell hybridisation and modelling methods.

7.1. GENEALOGICAL METHOD

The genealogical method is a method of studying pedigrees by means of which the distribution of a disease (trait) in a family or in an ancestor is traced, indicating the type of kinship between the members of the pedigree.

In medical genetics, the method is more commonly referred to as clinical genealogical, because it is the study of pathological traits in a family using clinical examination techniques. In contrast to morphological, immunological, biochemical and other special methods, which sometimes require complex equipment and long and painstaking laboratory analysis, the clinical genealogical method is relatively simple and accessible to every medical staff. At the same time, it can be used to obtain a lot of useful information, which will help to make the correct diagnosis, and, consequently, the prescription of adequate treatment and necessary preventive measures.

One of the main objectives of the clinical and genealogical method is:

1. Establishing the hereditary nature of the disease (trait) - this requires great care in collecting information about the relatives of the patient, remember the existence of the already mentioned phenocopies of hereditary diseases. For example, microcephaly in combination with mental retardation may be a consequence of a rare monogenic recessive mutation. At the same time, certain drugs taken by the mother during pregnancy or fetal X-rays may cause similar defects and represent a phenocopy of a genetically determined disease.
2. Determination of the type of inheritance of the disease (trait) - autosomal recessive, autosomal dominant, X-linked dominant or recessive.
3. Estimation of gene penetrance.
4. Timely diagnosis of hereditary diseases. Some diseases have a typical, easily identifiable clinical picture. Relatively common and therefore easily diagnosed (e.g. haemophilia, polydactyly, colour blindness), other diseases are rare, and for some there are only single descriptions in the world literature (e.g. it is difficult to diagnose the main forms of myopathy in the initial stages, myotonic dystrophy, Charcot-Marie neural amyotrophy).

The genealogical method is also widely used in medical genetic counselling, in particular to determine the prognosis of offspring in families where there is or is expected to be a patient with hereditary pathology. Two stages can be conditionally distinguished in the genealogical method: compilation of a pedigree and genealogical analysis.

Pedigree compilation. In this method, the collection of information about the family begins with the *proband*, the individual who is the subject of the doctor's study. Children of the same parental couple (siblings) are called sibs. If sibs have only one parent in common, they are called *half-sibs.* A distinction is made between half-sibs who share a half-sibling (common mother) and half-sibs who share a half-sibling (common father).

Usually a pedigree is collected on one or more traits. Most often the patient or counsellor is concerned about a particular disease or trait. The information is collected according to a specific pattern:

1. Anamnesis of the proband's present illness, its onset, its subsequent course, questioning about the patient's previous life;
2. Asking about the proband's sibs (birth order number, health status, etc.);
3. Asking about the closest relatives (first of all about the proband's parents). Next, the questioning of relatives on the mother's side begins. It is more convenient to record information in the following order: maternal grandmother and grandfather, their children in order of birth with indication of descendants (grandchildren). Information on stillbirths, miscarriages with indication of the cause, and infertile marriages is collected. Information on the relatives of the patient's father is collected in the same sequence.

All information about the proband should be collected in chronological order. It is important to find out what illnesses the child has had and how they have progressed. The assessment of all these points often makes the diagnosis much easier.

After data collection, it is necessary to proceed to the objective examination of the proband and his relatives, which consists of a detailed examination with description of phenotypic manifestations of the disease. Clinical examination of patients with hereditary pathology has great resolution. It is of particular importance because the correct diagnosis can often be established only by taking into account all the features of appearance.

When examining patients (probands), along with the detection of congenital malformations and anthropometry, attention should be paid to developmental microanomalies, or congenital morphogenetic variants. They are non-specific signs of embryonic dysmorphogenesis.

Here is a brief list of the main dysmorphies.

I. Examination of the head and face may reveal the following:

1) Changes in the size of the head: a decrease of 10% of the normal age range indicates microcephaly, an increase in the size of the head indicates macrocephaly. Hydrocephalus, or cerebral hydrocephalus, is characterised not only by an enlarged head but also by facial changes.

2) Anomalies of skull shapes: short broad skull vault, increase in the transverse diameter of the skull, the face is flattened - brachycephaly; tower skull - dolichocephaly; navicular shape of the head with a protruding forehead and occiput - scaphocephaly; triangular skull - trigonocephaly.

3) Hair: dry, sparse, woolly, grey strand above forehead, low hair growth on forehead and back of head.

4) Eye malformations: complete absence of one or both eyeballs - anophthalmos; absence of the eye slit, eyelids - ptosis; underdevelopment of the eyeball - cryptophthalmos; small eye size - microphthalmos; bull's eye - buphthalmos. Displacement of the eyeball forward - exophthalmos; displacement of the eyeball backwards - enophthalmos; drooping of the corners of the eyes (mongoloid eye section), etc.

5) Nose: saddle nose bridge, wide flat nose bridge, short nose, nostrils open forwards, flat nose wings, beak nose.

6) Lips and mouth: absence of jawbone - agnathia; forward or backward displaced upper jaws - prognathia and retrognathia; similar anomalies of the lower jaw - progenia and microgenia; cleft upper lip - cheiloschisis; enlargement and reduction of the mouth - macrostomia and microstomia, and of the tongue - macro and microglossia.

7) Teeth: enamel hypoplasia, irregular shape, malposition and excess of teeth, congenital absence of one or more teeth.

8) Sky: flat, high, arched, gothic.

9) Auricles: microtia, macrotia, deformed, low-lying, deviated backwards, protruding, preauricular papillomas.

10) Neck: short or long, low hair growth line, torticollis, wing folds.

II. Torso examination reveals absence - athelia and the presence of additional nipples - polythelia; overdevelopment of mammary glands in men - gynaecomastia; hernias of the white line of the abdomen, umbilical and inguinal-mastoid region. Deformities of the thorax and spine:

scoliosis, kyphosis, kyphoscoliosis.

III. When examining the ***limbs***, attention is paid to changes in their length as a whole and their individual parts: absence of a section or the whole limb - phocomelia; shortening of the limb - brachymelia; shortening of the fingers - brachydactyly; curvature of the fingers - clinodactyly; long fingers - arachnodactyly; fusion of the phalanges of the fingers - symphalangia; bony fusions - syndactyly.

IV. A careful examination of the skin and its appendages - hair and nails reveals: keratinisation of the skin - ichthyosis; changes in skin pigmentation - albinism; pigmented spots - nevi; increased dryness of the skin, increased sweating - hyperhidrosis; increased hairiness - hypertrichosis; complete absence of hair, eyebrows, eyelashes - atrichosis or alopecia. Graphical representation of pedigree.

To analyse and visualise the collected information, a graphical representation of the pedigree is used. For this purpose, standard symbols (Fig. 53) and examples are used. However, depending on the tasks, goals and peculiarities of the pedigree, the compiler can use his own designations with obligatory explanation under the figure. For explanation of principles of designation and drawing up of pedigrees we give two examples (Fig. 54,55). As it is visible from these figures, generations are designated by Roman numerals from top to bottom. Usually they are placed to the left of the pedigree.

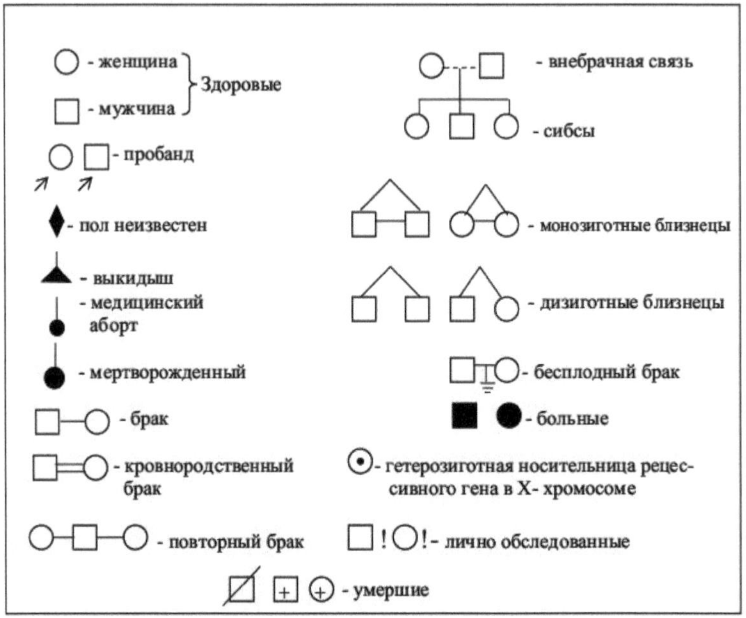

Figure 53. Symbols used in compiling a family tree.

The last generation of ancestors for which information has been collected is labelled as generation I. Arabic numerals number the offspring of one generation (the whole row) from left to right consecutively. Brothers and sisters are arranged in the genealogy in the order of birth (from the oldest to the youngest).

Thus, each member of the pedigree has its own cipher, e.g. II - 3, II - 5.

In cases where the spouse has not been investigated for the trait in question and his or her pedigree is not given, it is advisable not to depict him or her at all. All individuals of the same generation should be arranged strictly in one row, so it is preferable to draw the pedigree on lined paper. "Hanging" characters between rows of generations is a gross mistake. If the genealogy is very extensive, then different generations are not arranged in horizontal rows, but in concentric ones.

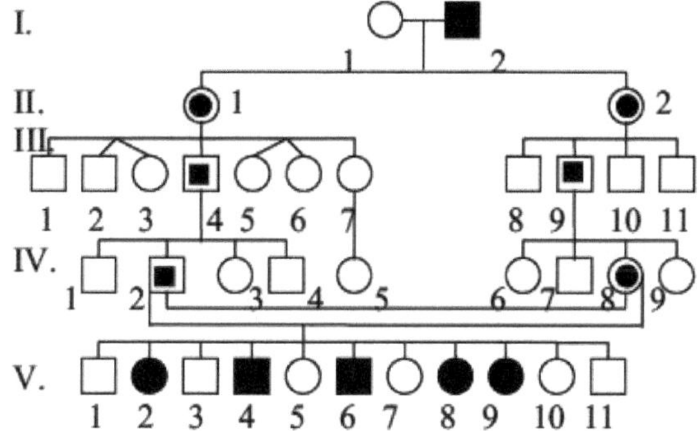

Figure 54 Pedigree with autosomal recessive type of inheritance of the disease, muscular dystrophy (Erb's progressive).

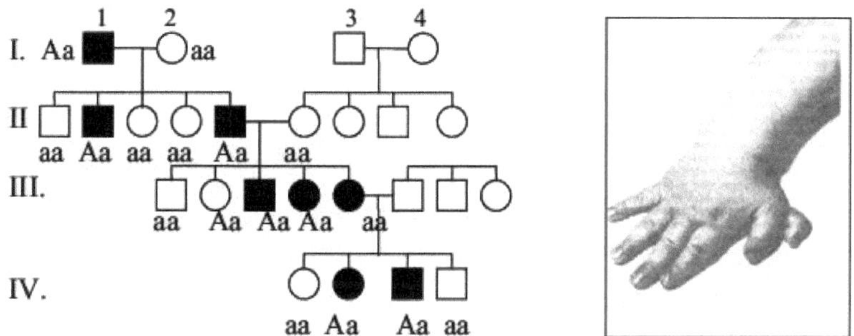

Figure 55. Pedigree with autosomal dominant type of inheritance of the polydactyly trait.

The graphic representation of the pedigree must be accompanied by a "pedigree legend", which is a mandatory element of the pedigree description and includes:

1) A description of the health status of a member of the pedigree, information about which is important for understanding the nature of inheritance of a disease (trait) or the peculiarities of its clinical manifestation;

2) The age of onset and the nature of the course of the disease in affected individuals;

3) The cause of death and age at death of the lineage member;

4) description of methods of diagnostics and identification of diseases, list of sources of medical and other information.

When applying the genealogical method, it is important to note in the pedigree of those personally examined for the presence of a trait (this can also be equated with obtaining information from an objective source, such as a medical history) and those not examined, information about whom is obtained from the answers of the proband or relatives, as well as from questionnaires. It is necessary to strive to obtain the most complete and objective primary material, which is the basis for statistical and genetic analyses and, consequently, the guarantee of the correctness and accuracy of the resulting conclusions.

Analysing the pedigree. Having carefully collected data on the pedigree, clarified the necessary information about the sick and examined the necessary family members, it is possible to start analysing the pedigree. In doing so, it is necessary to:

1) to determine whether the trait or disease is unique in the family or whether there are several cases of the pathology (familial);
2) Identify persons suspected of having the disease and plan for their examination and diagnosis;
3) Determine the type of inheritance and whether the disease is passed on through the maternal or paternal line;
4) to identify individuals in need of medical and genetic counselling, to determine the clinical prognosis for the proband and his or her ill relatives, taking into account the peculiarities of the disease and its genetic characteristics;
5) Develop a treatment and prevention plan, taking into account individual and family characteristics of the disease.

When analysing a pedigree, a physician may encounter gene and chromosomal diseases, diseases in the development of which both genetic and environmental factors are involved, and "unknown" diseases. Let us consider the main types of inheritance of monogenic diseases.

7.1.1. AUTOSOMAL DOMINANT TYPE OF INHERITANCE

Due to the fact that dominant genes determining the development of the disease are usually lethal in the homozygous state, all marriages between sick and healthy family members are of the type *Aa x aa*, where A is the dominant gene determining the development of the hereditary disease, and a is the recessive gene.

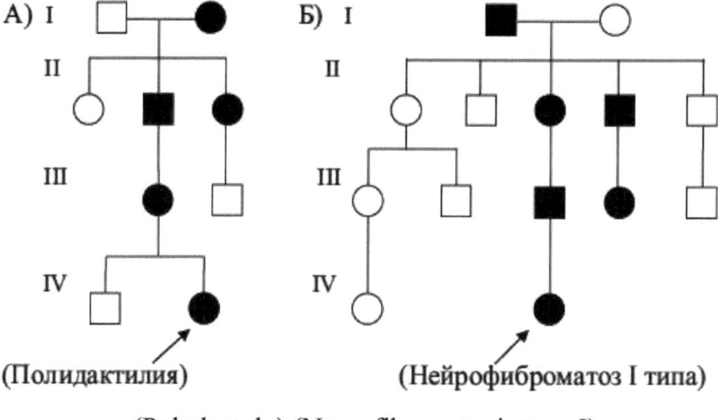

(Polydactyly) (Neurofibromatosis type I)

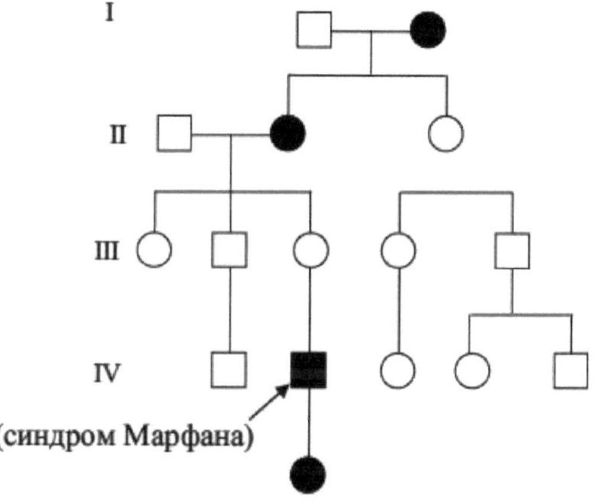

(Marfan syndrome)

Figure 56. An example of a pedigree:

A) Polydactyly of the classical autosomal dominant type.

B) Neurofibromatosis type I with autosomal dominant type of inheritance of expressive disease.

B) Marfan syndrome with autosomal dominant type of inheritance of the disease with incomplete penetrance.

The pedigree in this case has the following characteristic features:

1. Each sick family member usually has a sick parent.
2. The disease is transmitted from generation to generation; there are patients in every generation.
3. Healthy parents will have healthy children.
4. Both men and women can get the disease equally, as the gene is localised in the autosome.

5. The probability of having a sick child if one parent is sick is 50%.

Figure 56 shows the pedigree of a family "affected" by polydactyly (in the case of overaxial polydactyly, the extra finger is on the side of the first finger. In this case, there is a bifurcation of the I finger with duplication of all or part of its constituent elements). The anomaly is observed in every generation. From marriages where one of the spouses has such fingers and the other has normal fingers, children with the anomaly are born. This is one of the signs of dominant inheritance. The second sign that confirms the dominance of the gene is that from marriages where both parents have normal hand structure, there are no children with polydactyly. The anomaly is present to the same extent in both males and females. The above features are characteristic only for cases of the "classical" autosomal dominant type of inheritance. However, in practice, it is not uncommon for carriers of the dominant gene to remain phenotypically healthy, or their disease is of an erased nature. This can be explained by the fact that the gene for the disease has incomplete penetrance and one of the relatives does not appear (generation slippage), but he passed the gene to his son. For example, the disease, Huntington's chorea or Marfan syndrome are inherited with incomplete penetrance (Figure 56). A dominant gene has another property that makes it difficult to establish autosomal dominant inheritance. This is differential expressivity (the concept of expressivity is similar to the concept of disease severity). At very low gene expressivity, it seems that a person is healthy; at high expressivity, a severe form of the disease develops. For example, the disease neurofibromatosis.

To date, about 3000 autosomal dominant human traits have been described. The following monogenic diseases with autosomal dominant inheritance are the most common in clinical practice.

MARFAN SYNDROME

It is one of the hereditary forms of congenital generalised connective tissue pathology, first described in 1886.

The etiological factor of Marfan syndrome is a mutation in the fibrillin gene (localisation in chromosome 15 q). ***Marfan syndrome*** patients have a characteristic appearance: they are characterised by tall stature, asthenic physique, and a reduced amount of subcutaneous fat (Fig. 57),

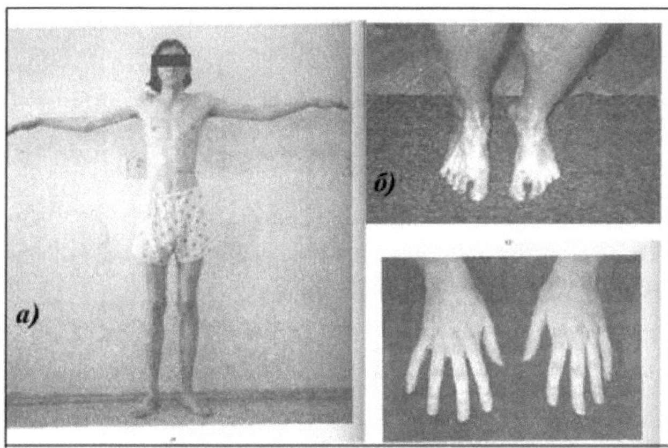

Figure 57. Marfan syndrome:
(a) Tall stature, asthenic build, arm span exceeding height (height 187 cm, arm span 193 cm);
b) "sandal-shaped shel" varicose veins of the lower leg;
c) arachnodactyly (long fingers).

The limbs are elongated mainly at the expense of distal parts, arm span exceeds the body length (in norm these parameters coincide). Long thin fingers are noted.

The "thumb symptom" is often observed, in which the long 1st finger of the hand in the transverse position reaches the ulnar edge of the narrow palm. When the 1st and 5th fingers cover the wrist of the other hand, they necessarily overlap. More than half of patients have chest deformity (funnel-shaped, wedge-shaped), curvature of the spine (kyphosis, scoliosis), hypermobility of joints, clinodactyly of little fingers, sandal-shaped cleft. On the part of the cardiovascular system the most pathognomonic are, dilation of the ascending part of the aortic arch with the development of aneurysms, prolapse of heart valves. On the part of visual organs the most characteristic are subluxations and dislocations of crystalline lens, retinal detachment, myopia, iris heterochromia. Half of patients have inguinal, umbilical and femoral hernias. Polycystic kidneys, hearing loss, deafness may be observed occasionally.

Mental and intellectual development of patients does not differ from the norm. The prognosis of life and health is determined primarily by the state of the cardiovascular system.

The average life expectancy for the severe form of Marfan syndrome is about 27 years, although some patients live to a ripe old age.

NEUROFIBROMATOSIS (RECKLINGHAUSEN'S DISEASE)

Seven nosological forms of ***neurofibromatosis*** are known, among which ***peripheral neurofibromatosis (type I)*** occupies the leading place.

It is one of the most common monogenic diseases. Currently, its genetics and clinical picture have been studied in detail. The gene for this disease has been fully decoded, more than 100 mutations have been found in it, and it is located on the 17th chromosome. More than half of the cases of the disease are the result of new mutations.

This disease is manifested from birth or in the first decade of life by the formation of "coffee-and-milk" type spots on the skin, which gradually increase in number and size (see Figure 45). As a rule, the spots are oval in shape, and they are usually located on closed areas of the skin - on the chest, back, and abdomen (five or more spots with a diameter of 0.5 cm in a child and six or more spots with a diameter of 1.5 cm in an adult suggest the diagnosis of neurofibromatosis).

As patients get older, small tumours (neurofibromas) appear on the skin, ranging from a few to several hundred. They can be localised everywhere, including the mucous membranes of the mouth and tongue. Patients with up to 10,000 or more neurofibromas have been described.

Neurofibromas are soft nodules that seem to fall into the skin when pressed - the "bell button" symptom. Subcutaneous nodules are located along the course of nerve trunks (rounded beads 1-2 cm in diameter, mobile, not attached to the skin). In addition, some patients develop diffuse massive tumour-like masses. Almost all patients have changes in the bone system - kyphosis, scoliosis, pseudoarthroses, local gigantism, non-specific craniofacial anomalies. Freckles in the axillary and inguinal folds, patchy hyperpigmentation of the skin of the upper chest and perineum are also frequent symptoms of this disease. In some cases, rarely in childhood, the tumours may become malignant.

Learning difficulties are observed in 30% of patients. Mental retardation is shallow and not progressive.

HOLT-ORAMA SYNDROME (HAND-HEART SYNDROME)

Holt-Oram syndrome is a monogenic syndrome of multiple congenital malformations. The clinical picture is characterised by anomalies of the upper limbs and congenital heart defects. Hand malformations range from hypo- or aplasia of the 1st finger, triphalangeal 1st finger of the hand (Figure 58) to hypo- and aplasia of the radius (radial club hand). The left hand is affected more often than not.

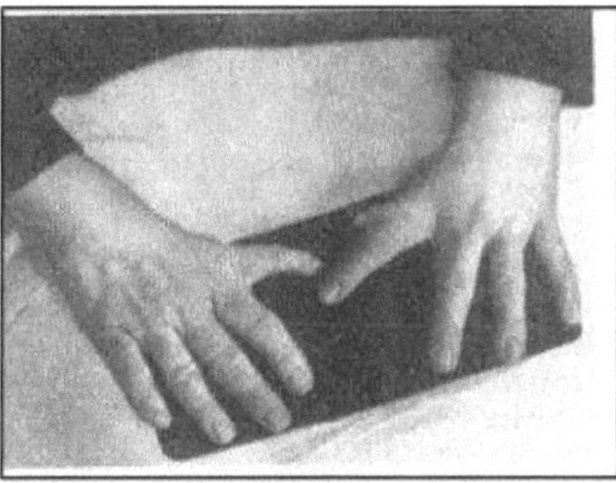

Figure 58. Holt-Oram syndrome.

Other skeletal changes are often observed: hypoplasia of the scapulae and clavicles, scoliosis, funnel-shaped deformity of the sternum, clinodactyly, syndactyly, hypoplasia of the hand and wrist bones. Congenital heart defects are not specific and manifest as defects of the interatrial and interventricular septum, open aortic duct, coarctation of the aorta, tetrada Fallo, pulmonary artery stenosis, mitral valve prolapse and others.

Relatives of patients should be carefully examined and examined due to the varying expression of the syndrome and the likelihood of detecting minimal manifestations of the pathological gene. Diagnosis is made on the basis of clinical and genealogical data and paraclinical examination. Prognosis of life depends on the severity of cardiac damage.

7.1.2. AUTOSOMAL RECESSIVE INHERITANCE

The main feature of a recessive gene is that it manifests its effect only in the homozygous state. Therefore, in the heterozygous state, it can exist in many generations without manifesting itself phenotypically.

As a result, the first patient with a recessive disease appears many generations after the mutation occurs, since a sick child can only be born if both parents carry the recessive disease gene.

There are three variants of such marriages:

1) ***aahaa*** - all children are sick (e.g. from the marriage of two albinos, all children will be albino);

2) ***Aa x aa*** - 50% of the children will be sick (aa), 50% will be phenotypically healthy (Aa) but will carry the mutant gene;

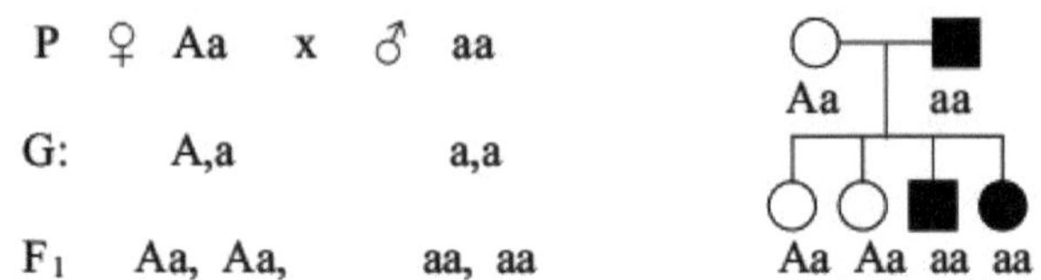

3) ***Aa x Aa*** - 25% of the children will be sick (Aa), 75% will be phenotypically healthy (AA and Aa), but 50% of them (Aa) will be carriers of the pathological gene.

Autosomal recessive inheritance has the following distinguishing features:

1. Sick children are born to healthy parents. The most common type of marriage is between heterozygous carriers (Aa x Aa), where both parents are phenotypically healthy but may have children with a homozygous genotype.
2. Healthy children are born to a sick parent. When a sick person with a recessive disease marries a healthy person (AA x aa), all children will be healthy.
3. Sibs (brothers, sisters), not parents - children, as in the dominant type of inheritance.
4. The pedigree shows a higher percentage of consanguineous marriages (see Figure 54).
5. All parents of sick children are heterozygous carriers of the pathological gene.
6. Men and women are equally likely to get the disease.
7. In heterozygous carriers, the ratio of sick to healthy children is 1:3. The probability of giving birth to a sick child is 25% for each subsequent child.

In autosomal recessive inheritance, as in autosomal dominant inheritance, different degrees of expression and penetrance rates are possible.

MUCOVISCIDOSIS (PANCREATIC CYSTOFIBROSIS)

The disease is caused by generalised damage to the exocrine glands. The incidence of ***cystic fibrosis*** among newborns in European populations is 1:2500. At the same time, the disease is rare in eastern populations and in African black populations (1:100000). The cystic fibrosis gene is localised on chromosome 7. About 1000 mutations have been found in it, about 300 of which cause clinical manifestations. The gene determines the synthesis of a protein called cystic fibrosis transmembrane conductance regulator.

The pathogenesis of the disease is due to the fact that in the absence of synthesis of the primary gene product (transmembrane regulator), chloride transport in epithelial cells is impaired. This leads to excessive chloride excretion, which results in hypersecretion of thick mucus in the cells of the exocrine part of the pancreas, bronchial epithelium, and the mucous membrane of the gastrointestinal tract. Exhaust ducts of the pancreas are blocked, mucus is not excreted, cysts are formed. Pancreatic enzymes do not enter the intestinal lumen.

Hyperproduction of mucus in the bronchial tree leads to blockage of small bronchi and subsequent adherence of infection. Similar processes develop in the sinuses of the nose and in the tubules of the testes. There is an increased concentration of sodium and chlorine ions in sweat fluid, which is the main diagnostic laboratory test.

The following clinical forms of the disease are distinguished: mixed (pulmonary-intestinal 65-75% of all patients); predominantly pulmonary (15-20%); predominantly intestinal (5-10%); meconial ileus (not more than 1%); sterile and abortive forms (insignificant proportion). In practice, mixed forms of the disease are the most common.

The first symptoms of the disease appear in the first year of life, usually against the background of acute respiratory viral infection and are characterised by an attack-like compulsive cough, obstruction and inflammation of the lungs. Recurrent chronic infectious-inflammatory process is complicated by purulent obstructive bronchitis, pneumonia, occurring several times a year. Secondary changes include bronchiectasis, emphysema, 185
pneumosclerosis, pulmonary heart disease. In parallel, patients have symptoms of the gastrointestinal tract. Digestive disorders are manifested by impaired weight gain, abdominal bloating, profuse smelly stools with an admixture of fat. Appetite in children is preserved.

Subsequently, the liver is involved in the pathological process (fatty infiltration, cholestatic hepatitis, cirrhosis).

Meconium ileus is a congenital form of the disease, manifested in the first day after birth by the absence of meconium discharge and the clinic of complete intestinal obstruction. Intellectual development in children is not affected. Life prognosis in all forms of cystic fibrosis, except typical forms, is unfavourable.

Currently, patients with mixed forms rarely live more than 20 years.

7.1.3. X - LINKED TYPE OF INHERITANCE

Genes localised in the *X* chromosome, as well as in autosomal inheritance, can be dominant and recessive. The main feature of *the X-linked* type of inheritance is the absence of transmission of the corresponding gene from father to son, since men, being *hemizygous* (having only one *X* chromosome*)*, pass their X chromosome *only to* their daughters.

If a dominant gene is localised in chromosome *X*, this type of inheritance is called^-linked dominant inheritance.

It is characterised by the following features:

1. If a father is sick, all his daughters will be sick and all his sons will be healthy.
2. Children will only be sick if one parent is sick.
3. With healthy parents, all children will be healthy.
4. The disease can be traced back to every generation.
5. If the mother is sick, the probability of having a sick child is equal, 50% independent of gender.
6. Both men and women get sick, but in general there are twice as many sick women in the family as sick men.

Analysis of the pedigree shown in (Fig. 59) shows that the trait of brown tooth enamel colouration is inherited by dominant type. This is evidenced by the fact that children with brown teeth are born from marriages in which one parent is sick and the other is healthy (Figure 59-1).

If the mother is heterozygous and inherits the disease and the father is healthy, the probability of having sick children is 50% regardless of sex (Figure 59-2).

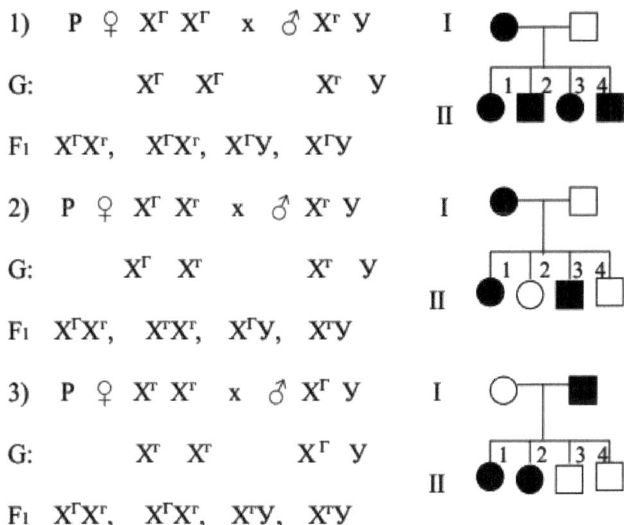

Figure 59. Pedigree of a family with brown tooth enamel colouration.

If the mother has white teeth and the father has brown teeth, then only the males of that generation will have normal enamel colouration and all females will inherit the enamel colouration defect (Figure 59-3).

When a recessive gene is localised in chromosome *X,* the type of inheritance is called U-linked recessive.

This type is characterised by the following:

1. The disease predominantly affects males.
2. The disease is seen in male maternal relatives of the proband.
3. A son never inherits his father's disease.
4. If the proband is a woman, her father is necessarily sick, and all her sons are also sick.
5. From the marriage of sick men and healthy women, all children will be healthy, but daughters may have sick sons.
6. A marriage between a healthy man and a heterozygous woman has a 50% chance of producing a sick child for boys and 0% for girls.

The pedigree shown in Figure 60 shows that only males have the disease. This suggests that the disease gene is sex-linked. As a rule, sick children are born to healthy parents. At the same time, children from marriages of sick men with healthy women are healthy regardless of sex.

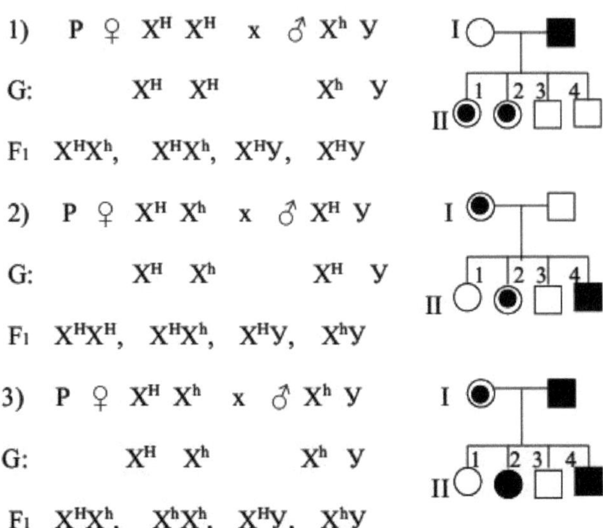

Figure 60. Pedigree of a family with haemophilia.

This is possible when the recessive gene for the disease is located in chromosome *X*, In males, chromosome *X is* only one and the recessive gene cannot be suppressed. Women, on the other hand, have two chromosomes .V.

Therefore, if a woman inherits this *X* chromosome *with the* disease gene from her father, the dominant norm gene of the other *X* chromosome from her mother will "suppress" the disease gene.

PSEUDOHYPERTROPHIC DUCHENNE MUSCULAR DYSTROPHY

It is one of the most frequent forms of inherited neuromuscular diseases. It was first described in 1868. Muscular dystrophies

characterised by degenerative changes in the transverse striated muscles without primary peripheral motoneuron pathology. Its incidence is 1:3000-1:5000 boys.

The disease is caused by a disorder in the synthesis of the protein dystrophin. The dystrophin gene is localised in the short arm of the X chromosome and has been cloned and sequenced. It is the longest gene studied.

The main symptomatology of the disease lies in the progressive increase of muscular dystrophic changes with gradual immobilisation of the patient. In children under three years of age, it is quite difficult to diagnose the disease. It is known that these children somewhat lag behind in motor development in the first year of life - they start sitting and walking later.

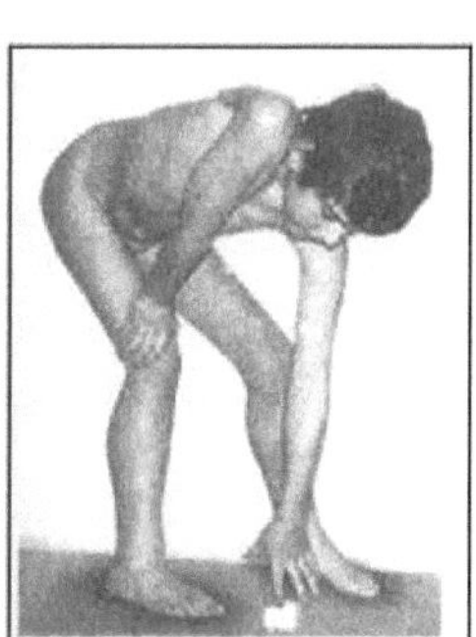
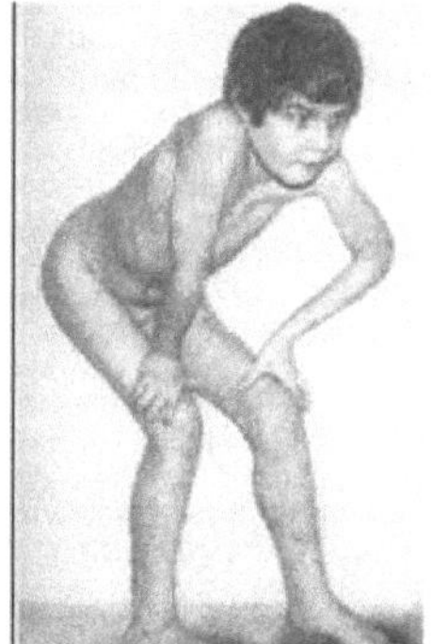

Figure 61. Duchenne muscular dystrophy.

Never running or jumping.

The classic picture of the disease appears in children of three to five years of age. One of the first signs is a thickening of the calf muscles and a gradual increase in their volume due to the growth of connective and fatty tissue. Already at an early stage of the disease, children have difficulty getting up from the floor, from "squatting". From a forward bent position, the child rises "on its own" (Fig. 61). Atrophy of the thigh and pelvic girdle muscles is often masked by well-developed subcutaneous fatty tissue. Gradually, the process takes an upward direction and spreads to the shoulder girdle, back muscles and then to the proximal arms. In the terminal stage, muscle weakness

can spread to the muscles of the face, neck, pharynx.

In the advanced stage of the disease there are such characteristic symptoms as a "duck-like" gait, pronounced lumbar lordosis, wing-shaped shoulder blades. Early muscle contractures are typical. Pseudohypertrophies can also develop in the gluteal and deltoid muscles of the tongue and abdomen. Very often the heart muscle is affected, heart rhythm disturbances, dilated heart borders, ECG changes are detected. Acute heart failure is the most frequent cause of death. Approximately 50% of children have a decrease in intelligence - from borderline conditions to pronounced debility. Patients die, as a rule, in the third decade of life, and by 14-15 years of age, they are usually immobile.

7.2. TWIN METHOD

Twins are born about 1% of the time, hence they make up about 2% of all newborns. Twins are of two types. *Dizygotic*, or *identical, twins* develop from two different eggs fertilised simultaneously by different sperm.

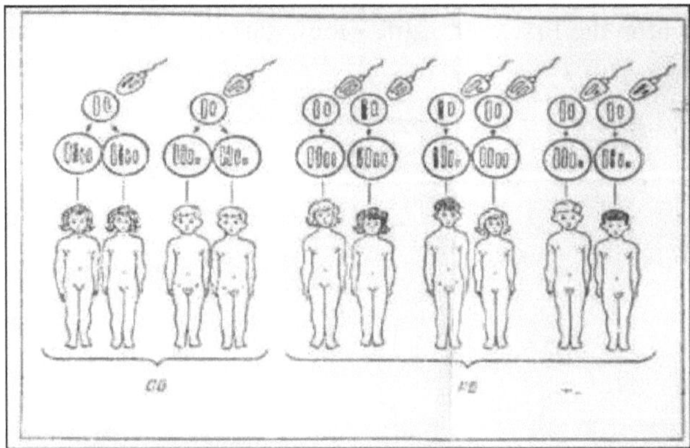

Figure 62. Monozygotic and dizygotic twins.

Thus, the main reason for the birth of dizygotic twins is the simultaneous ovulation, in their mothers of two eggs. Dizygotic twins can be either of the same or different sexes, and their ratio looks like: 1($+$) : 2($+^) : 1($+$). Identical twins are no more genetically similar than normal siblings. The frequency of birth of identical twins depends on the age of the mother, her genotype and environmental factors.

Sometimes one fertilised egg gives rise to not one, but two (or more) embryos. *Monozygotic,* or *identical, twins* develop from them. They are always of the same sex: either boys or girls, in approximately equal proportions (Figure 62). The similarity of monozygotic twins is very high because they share the same genotype. Identical twins are of interest for studying the interaction between genotype and environmental factors, since the differences between them are mainly due to the influence of developmental conditions, i.e. the external environment. The proportion of identical twins in humans is about 35-38% of the total number of twins.

Establishing the type of twins is not always easy. It is possible to rule out monozygosity accurately, but it is much more difficult and not always possible to prove it. For this purpose, such signs as blood group, various serum proteins and enzymes are used. A reliable, though difficult to apply technique in resolving this issue is skin grafting. In monozygotic twins, reciprocal skin grafts are completed successfully, while in dizygotic twins skin grafts are rejected.

In 1876, the English researcher F. Galton proposed to use the method of twin analysis to distinguish the influence of heredity and environment on the development of various traits in humans.

The essence of this method consists of two variants of comparisons: comparison of pairs of identical twins with same-sex identical twins, as well as comparison of pairs of identical twins raised together and separately. If the trait under study appears in both twins, it is called *concordance*, if only one of them, it is called *discordance.*

For example, according to blood type, a couple is considered concordant if both partners have the same blood type, but if the blood type of the partners is different, the couple is discordant. To prove the role of heredity in the development of a trait, it is enough to compare the proportion (percentage) of concordant pairs in groups of mono- and dizygotic twins.

Let's consider this on the example of diabetes mellitus. If one of the monozygotic twins has diabetes, the second partner gets the disease in 65% of cases (in 65% of cases they are concordant). If one of the dizygotic twins has diabetes, the second partner has diabetes only 18% of the time. The large concordance in the group of genetically identical partners of monozygotic pairs proves that hereditary predisposition plays a significant role in the etiology of diabetes. Various formulae are used to quantify the role of heredity and environment. The most commonly used are the coefficients of heritability (H) and environmental influence (E), calculated according to the Holzinger formula:

$$H = \frac{C_{mz} - C_{dz}}{100 - C_{dz}} \cdot 100 \;; \quad E = 100 - H,$$

where C_{mz} *is the* percentage of concordant pairs in the group of monozygotic twins, and C_{dz} *is the* same in the group of dizygotic twins. In the above example of diabetes mellitus, the proportion of hereditary causation of the trait is:

$$H = \frac{65 - 18}{100 - 18} \cdot 100 = 57\%,$$

and the influence of the environment $E = 100 - 57 = 43\%$. Results

calculations using Holzinger's formulae confirm that diabetes is due to genetic factors as much as environmental conditions.

Let us use Holzinger's formula in two more examples. Suppose that a trait (blood type) is entirely determined by genotype and does not depend on environmental influences. In this case in a group of monozygotic twins the concordance of the partners is complete due to the identity of their genotypes (C_{mz} = 100%), while the concordance in a group of dizygotic twins, determined by a random combination of their parents' genes, will be incomplete, for example: 40% (C_{dz} = 40%). Substituting these values into Holzinger's formula, we obtain:

$$H = \frac{100-40}{100-40} \cdot 100 = 100\%; \; E = 0\%.$$

A different result is obtained for a trait, the development of which does not depend on genotype and is completely determined by the influence of the environment (this is the case with some infectious diseases). In this case, the percentage of concordant pairs in groups of mono- and dizygotic twins is the same, for example, 90% in both groups. Substituting these values of concordance into Holzinger's formula, we get H=0%, *E*= 100%. Consequently, the coefficient of inheritability for different traits is different; it varies from 100% for traits completely determined by genetic factors to 0% for traits entirely dependent on environmental influences. In most cases, the development of traits is determined by the joint influence of genotype and environmental conditions, then the coefficient of heritability is less than 100% and more than 0%, and it is the greater the stronger the influence of the genetic factor.

The coefficient of heritability can also be calculated for quantitative traits in which the partners of a pair differ from each other not by the alternative "concordants-discordants", but by the expression of the trait. In these cases, the coefficient of heritability is calculated using a slightly modified Holzinger formula:

$$H = \frac{r_{mz} - r_{dz}}{1 - r_{dz}} \cdot 100 \; ; \qquad E = 100 - H,$$

where r_{mz} *is the* intraclass correlation coefficient in the group of monozygotic twins, and r_{dz} *is the* same in the group of dizygotic twins.

The mathematical apparatus of twin analysis has been considerably expanded in recent years, which makes it possible in some cases to obtain additional information about the relative importance of genotype and environment in the ontogenesis of organism traits.

Thus, traits characterised by a high level of concordance are largely or predominantly determined by genetic factors and are little confirmed by the influence of environmental conditions. Traits characterised by high discordance, on the contrary, are mainly determined by the influence of the environment.

It should not be thought that monozygotic twins should always be absolutely similar to each other in qualitative features. The cause of differences may be somatic cell mutations and variations in gene expression at all stages of development, including the earliest stages. An example is the description of monozygotic sisters with a normal karyotype, one of whom had haemophilia and the other was a heterozygous carrier of the haemophilia gene with no signs of the disease. The discordance between the sisters was probably due to the fact that early developmental inactivation of the *X chromosome* was different in them.

The use of the twin method confirms the important conclusion that any trait of the human organism is the result of the action of genes and environmental conditions.

7.3. CYTOGENETIC METHODS

The study of the structure and function of chromosomes has led to the isolation of an independent section of science - *cytogenetics.* The beginning of the development of human cytogenetics can be considered to be the 50-60s, when for the first time there appeared publications of works in which it was possible to obtain convincing pictures of the morphology of all human chromosomes and correctly determine their diploid number.

The essence of cytogenetic methods with all the variety of individual stages is in the microscopic analysis of chromosomes, allowing to detect numerical and structural changes in the chromosomal set (karyotype), the so-called chromosomal and genomic mutations.

Cytogenetic techniques are widely incorporated into medicine. It has been found that multiple malformations in newborns are often due to chromosomal abnormalities. A significant proportion of chromosomal and genomic mutations have been detected in stillborn and spontaneously aborted embryos. Cytogenetics of human malignant tumours has also started to develop. Thus, cytogenetics is now firmly embedded in the practice of public health. Cytogenetic research methods can be conditionally subdivided into *direct and indirect.*

Direct methods are methods of obtaining preparations of dividing cells without culturing. This method allows chromosomal analysis of tumour cells, but is mainly used for bone marrow studies. Bone marrow is obtained by sternal puncture, placed in nutrient medium, colchicine is added (it stops cell division at the metaphase stage of mitosis), cells are incubated for about 2-3 h at 37^0 C, and then chromosome preparations are prepared.

Indirect methods are the preparation of chromosome preparations from cells cultured in artificial nutrient media. Chromosome preparations can be prepared from all tissues and cell suspensions containing dividing cells. In humans, preparations from bone marrow cells, short-term blood culture or long-term fibroblast culture are used in most cases.

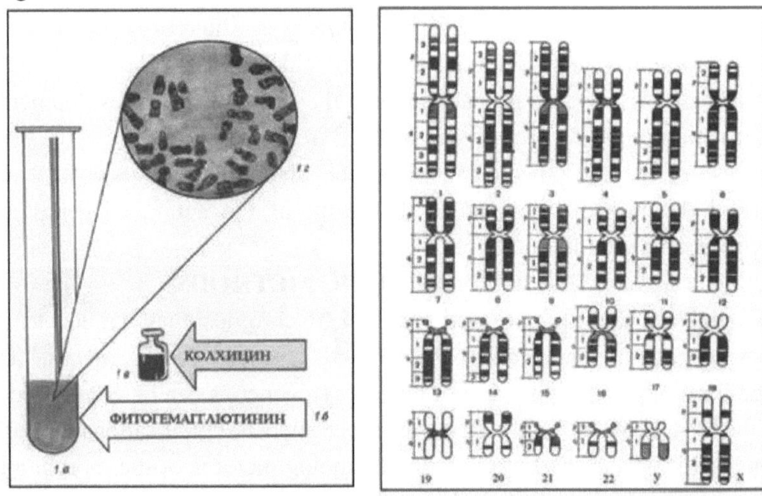

Figure 63. Human chromosome staining by differential staining with Giemsa dye and schematic representation of chromosome loci.

The blood cell culture method is the easiest and most accessible. Bone marrow puncture or skin biopsy to culture fibroblasts is technically more difficult and also a very unpleasant procedure. Indirect methods involve culturing cells. There are no dividing cells in the blood of healthy people (or patients, but not leukaemia). However, mitosis of these cells can be stimulated artificially. For this purpose, blood obtained in an amount of 1.0 ml is used. The blood is placed in nutrient medium with the addition of the mitogen FHA (phytohaemagglutinin), which stimulates mitotic division of lymphocytes. The culture is then placed in a thermostat and cultured for 48-72 h at 37^0 C. Colchicine is administered 2 h before the end of cultivation (Fig. 63).

Fibroblast culture is obtained from skin biopsy material. It is crushed and grown in culture medium so that the pieces are attached to the surface of the culture vessel. After 10 days the cells start to grow on this surface, after 21 days the suspension is prepared and preparations are made.

A very important point for the analysis of chromosomes is their staining. Solid or uniform staining of chromosomes is called *routine staining.*

Simple dyes are used for routine staining: Gimza or 2% acetoorsein or 2% acetocarmine. These dyes stain the whole chromosomes, uniformly and intensely. For some diagnostic purposes (for example, for the detection of numerical anomalies of chromosomes) this method is quite sufficient. To obtain a more detailed picture of the chromosome structure and to identify individual chromosomes or their segments, different methods of differential staining are used.

Cytogenetic methods immediately found practical application in the diagnosis of chromosomal diseases. For example, a married couple who had been married for 3 years came for infertility counselling. The wife was observed in the women's clinic for three years and received intensive therapy for infertility. The husband was not examined. When the husband was examined by a geneticist, Klinefelter syndrome was suspected. A cytogenetic study of the karyotype confirmed the doctor's diagnosis. His chromosome set is 47, XXU. This chromosomal pathology was the cause of infertility.

A relatively recent addition to the arsenal of laboratory cytogenetics are high-resolution methods - the *molecular cytogenetic method of in situ hybridisation,* in particular fluorescence *in situ* hybridisation or *FISH* - method.

FISH method is based on the treatment of chromosome preparations with a specific DNA probe, which is attached to the chromosome under study, and after treatment with special compounds and fluorescent dyes, the preparation is examined using a fluorescent microscope. To compare the resolving power of the method we give the following information. In routine chromosome staining, the smallest broken section of a chromosome in the form of a deletion or duplication, which can be distinguished under an ordinary light microscope, contains $30 \cdot 10^6$ nucleotides.

The use of differential staining methods increases this possibility to $(7-10) \cdot 10^6$ nucleotides. When analysing chromosomes at the stage of early metaphase or prophase, microrearrangements of $(1-3) \cdot 10^6$ nucleotides are distinguishable. The next level of resolution is provided only by the molecular cytogenetic method. Such a high resolution of the method allows to apply directly FISH - method or its variants in a wide enough range: from determination of gene localisation to deciphering of complex chromosome rearrangements.

Thus, cytogenetic methods have become practically indispensable procedures in various fields of science and clinical practice. In addition to disease diagnosis, cytogenetic methods are widely used in preventive medicine.

7.4. DERMATOGLYPHIC TESTING

American scientists C. Cummis and C. Midlo at the beginning of the century stated about the possible use of ***dermatoglyphics*** to identify the genetic features of the human body and its predisposition to various diseases.

The name *"dermatoglyphics"* (from Greek *derma* - skin, *gliphica* - to engrave)" was proposed by them and introduced into science. The study of skin patterns began from ancient times, Malpighi (1686) and Purkinje (1823) in their works on anatomy gave types of skin patterns. The study of skin patterns is one of the most convenient and accessible methods of revealing genetic features of the human organism.

It is believed that dermatoglyphic traits are more stable over time and more reliably indicate the persistence of ancient population traits.

Since the late 50s of this century, research in the field of dermatoglyphics has been widely developed. The method of dermatoglyphics is widely used in medical research to identify predisposition to diseases, the nature of their course and causes. The use of dermatoglyphic testing of pre-school children allowed to identify among them a group of increased risk for bronchopulmonary diseases and, to a certain extent, to predict the features of their course. Eastern medicine believes that the shape, size of hands and fingers, as well as the configuration of the main lines can serve as a key to determining the general state of health of patients, as well as his psychological state and establishing the diagnosis of the disease.

To date, 36 consistent features have been described, a set of which can be used to draw conclusions about the presence of a particular congenital pathology, some of which are summarised below:

Features of dermatoglyphic pattern in various diseases

Disease	Dermatoglyphic features	Author, year
Schizophrenia	In women and men, the total crest count (TCC) is decreased, the atd angle is increased, and the relative frequency of individual patterned types on the fingers is altered. In females, the frequency of carthoral loops on the hypothenor is decreased, and the frequency of dysplasias is increased on the left hand. In males, the frequency of patterns on the 3rd	**Michelsar, 1977**

	interfinger pad and the frequency of transverse folds on the right hand is increased, and dysplasias are observed.	
Oligophrenia **Oligophrenia**	The total comb count of OGS (right+left hands) is equal to 154.3±3.3 and 144.5±4.4 combs in female and male oligrophenics, 141.5±3.9 and 149.7±5.2 combs in controls, 171.5±6.5 and 139.5±8.8 combs in the group of imbeciles and idiots. Pattern count in oligophrenia by loops and whorls in males 13.45±0.11 and 20.35±0.13, in females 13.15±0.20 and 19.50±0.21 crests, in controls in males 13.50±0.20 and 20.00±0.304, in controls in females 13.00±0.22 and 18.05±0.25. There was an increase in crest count in male oligophrenics and a decrease in female oligophrenics.	**Ritzner et al, 1972** **Ritzner et al, 1972**
Down syndrome	The main palm lines end in regions with higher numerical values, the axial t triradius is located higher, the angle atd is larger, the frequency of the pattern on the hypotenor is higher in the main ulnar direction, in the ulnar direction	**Trepakov, 1989**
	shifted patterns on the fingertips, and in the middle phalanges of the fingers below normal, the little finger is shortened.	
Ischaemic heart disease	1. Increased the number of ulnar loops (more than half). 2. Absence of curls. 3. Termination of line A in the 5th field. 4. Increased patterning of the III and IV interfinger spaces. 5. Increased patterning of the hypotenor. 6. proximal location of the axial triradius G. 7. Presence of additional axial triradiuses and position t and t".	**Chistikin, 1995**
Neuroses	Patients have a lower total crest count (TCC), a greater frequency of hypotenor patterns, women with TCC>164 and men >170 are less prone to neurosis than individuals with low TCC (111 and 118 crests) and medium (112-163) for women and medium (119-169) for men.	**Michelsar, 1977**

The subject of study of dermatoglyphologists is ridged skin, which is present only on the palm surfaces of the hands and the plantar surfaces of the feet. The dermatoglyphic method of study is based on the anatomy, embryogenesis and genetics of skin patterns (Fig. 64).

Figure 64. Dactyloscopy.

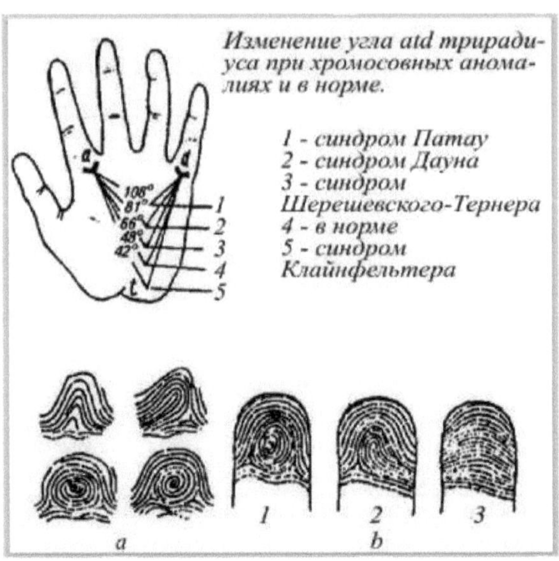

As it is known, the human skin consists of two main layers: the outer *epidermis* and the *skin* itself *(dermis).* The skin of the palm surface of hands, fingers and the plantar surface of the human foot has morphological features different from other covering structures. The papillary layer is well developed in the dermis of these skin areas. Coming to the surface, the papillae form elevations in the form of scallops called papillary lines. Epidermis, covering the rows of papillae of the dermis, forms a peculiar surface relief. Each papilla occupies a permanent place in the dermis, which predetermines the character of the relief of papillary lines. They are arranged mainly in papillary rows, which can form different patterns: *arcs (arch) - A, loops (loop) - L* and *whorls (whorl) - W.* Papillary lines are separated from each other by depressions (grooves) 1.2 to 0.4 μm wide. Apart from fine papillary engraving, the surface of the fingers of palms and feet is riddled with deeper flexion folds or flexion furrows (thumb flexion, distal and proximal).

It should be emphasised that the scallop skin is formed in the fetal period from the 12th week to the 6th month of intrauterine development. According to the orientation of the loop pattern on the surface of the finger pad, the patterns are distinguished as ulnar and radial (the curve of the thumb is ulnar, opposite is radial). The type and orientation does not change with age. Such quantitative index of dermatoglyphics as crest count does not change either. Crest score is a stable, not changing with age feature of finger dermatoglyphics. Ridge width - ridge and furrow width, like the size of the central pattern fragment, changes with age. However, both crest width and the size of the central fragment of the pattern are primary morphogenetic structures of scalloped skin.

It is characteristic that, at each race of the person patterns on fingers have a specific drawing of patterns. Russians, Ukrainians and Belarusians have very similar patterns on their fingers and speak about common origin. But each person has an individual pattern pattern and does not resemble others.

7.5. BIOCHEMICAL METHODS

Biochemical indicators reflect the essence of hereditary disease more accurately than clinical symptoms. Biochemical diagnosis assesses the phenotype of the organism at the molecular level, and hereditary disease is ultimately the phenotype. Therefore, biochemical methods have a leading role in the diagnosis of many monogenic diseases. However, the difficulty of diagnosis lies in the fact that hundreds of hereditary diseases by some biochemical indicators of urine or blood may be similar (e.g., acidosis, proteinuria, etc.). It is very time consuming and expensive to determine for each patient many metabolites. Knowledge of the general characteristics of metabolic changes in different hereditary diseases has allowed a new initial examination scheme to be constructed based on the clinical picture of the disease, genealogical information and biochemical analysis plan. This approach allows screening based on stepwise exclusion of certain classes of diseases (sieving methods).

Biochemical diagnosis of hereditary diseases uses both classical biochemical methods (electrophoresis, chromatography, spectroscopy) and modern high-precision technologies such as liquid chromatography, mass spectrometry, magnetic resonance spectrometry, and fast neutron bombardment. Biochemical examination of the patient allows identification of any metabolites specific to the hereditary disease suspected of which the patient has been referred. Each examination should begin with a plan based on clinical and genetic information about the patient and his or her family. The "objects" of biochemical diagnosis are biological fluids: urine, sweat, blood plasma and serum, red blood cells, leukocytes, cultures of fibroblasts, lymphocytes.

In almost all cases, biochemical diagnosis begins with a *screening* approach, in which two levels are distinguished: primary and clarifying. The primary level of diagnosis is to exclude healthy individuals from further examination. Two types of primary biochemical diagnosis are distinguished: *mass and selective.* In the first stage, urine and blood are used.

There are ***mass screening programmes for*** the diagnosis among newborns of phenylketonuria, congenital hypothyroidism, congenital adrenal hyperplasia, cystic fibrosis, galactosemia. The biological material for diagnosis is blood. Dried drops of capillary blood of newborns on chromatographic or filter paper are sent from maternity hospitals to the laboratory. The material should reach the laboratory within two to three days after sample collection.

To diagnose phenylketonuria, blood is taken from newborns in the maternity hospital on the 3rd to 5th day after birth. If the blood is taken earlier, false results are possible. In the laboratory, the amount of phenylalanine is determined by the following methods: microbiological test Guthrie, fluorometry, thin-layer chromatography and others. Experience has shown that missed cases are not errors in laboratory tests, but the result of negligence in the work of nurses when taking blood in maternity hospitals. In case of a positive result for phenylketonuria, a clarifying biochemical diagnosis is carried out by quantitative determination of phenylalanine in the blood.

Congenital hypothyroidism (decreased thyroid function) is also performed after the third day of life of the newborn, whether there is no decrease in plasma thyroxine levels and whether the thyroid hormone content of the pituitary gland is increased. In practice, two methods of sieving diagnosticsshdododioimmune *or immunoenzymatic* are used. These methods are approximately the same, but the enzyme immunoassay method is preferable, although it is more expensive.

Screening programmes for mass diagnoses of inherited diseases are not only for newborns. They can be organised to detect diseases that are common in certain populations or populations. For example, Jews have a high incidence of Tay-Sachs disease.

In the USA, a screening biochemical programme has been set up to detect heterozygosity for this disease, followed by medical and genetic counselling of such families. Thalassaemia, a severe blood disorder, occurs with high frequency in Italy. The health authorities in these countries have organised biochemical screening of the population to identify latent thalassaemia carriers (heterozygotes).

Selective diagnostic programmes involve checking biochemical metabolic abnormalities (urine, blood) in patients in whom gene inherited diseases are suspected. In fact, such programmes should operate in every large hospital. The indications for their use are quite broad. Selective programmes may use simple qualitative reactions (e.g. iron chloride test for phenylketonuria) or more precise methods that detect large groups of abnormalities. For example, thin-layer chromatography of urine and blood can be used to diagnose inherited disorders of amino acid, lipid and carbohydrate metabolism.

Gas chromatography is used to detect hereditary diseases of organic acid metabolism. Haemoglobin electrophoresis is used to diagnose the whole group of haemoglobinopathies. In modern conditions very many stages of biochemical diagnostics are carried out by automatic devices (amine analysers).

An example of a programme of selective screening for hereditary metabolic diseases with acute course and early lethal outcome is the programme developed by N.V. Zhukova at the Medical and Genetic Research Centre of the Russian Academy of Medical Sciences. This programme allows to detect 140 hereditary metabolic diseases in children.

Indications for the use of biochemical diagnostic methods in newborns are such symptoms as convulsions, coma, vomiting, hypotonia, jaundice, specific odour of urine and sweat, acidosis, disturbed acid-base balance, growth arrest. In children, biochemical methods are used in all cases of suspected hereditary metabolic diseases (delayed physical and mental development, loss of acquired functions, clinical picture specific to a hereditary disease).

7.6. POPULATION STATISTICAL METHOD

Population genetics studies the genetic structure of populations, their gene pool, factors and regularities that determine its preservation and change during the succession of generations. In medical genetics, the population method is used to study: hereditary diseases, patterns of their distribution, occurrence of pathological genotypes and genes in populations of different places, countries and cities. The study of the peculiarities of hereditary diseases distribution in connection with population structure also makes it possible to predict the prevalence of these diseases in subsequent generations.

By knowing the frequency of a trait or disease, it is possible to establish the genetic structure and gene pool of a population for that trait. The population structure is characterised by the frequency of genotypes controlling alternative variations of a trait, while the gene pool is characterised by the frequency of alleles of a given locus. In this connection, it is necessary first of all to familiarise ourselves with the concept of "frequency" and the ways of its expression.

The frequency of a particular genotype in a population is the relative number of individuals possessing that genotype. The frequency can be expressed as a percentage of the total number of individuals in the population, which is taken as 100%. More often in population genetics, the total number of individuals is taken as one. In this case, the frequency of a particular genotype is expressed in fractions of a unit.

If the entire population cannot be studied, a portion of the population is examined and the frequency is expressed as a percentage of the population.

For example, the MN-system blood type consists of three genotypes: $L^M L^M$, $L^N L^N$ AND $L^M L^N$. Genotype $L^M L^M$ is manifested by the presence of M antigen, genotype L $L^{N N}$ is manifested by the presence of N antigen. Genotype $L^M L^N$ is manifested by the presence of both antigens - (M,N) due to the codominance of alleles. Suppose that when determining MN - blood group in the population it is found that out of 4200 people examined 1218 people have only M antigen, 882 people have only N antigen and 2100 people have both antigens. It is required to determine the frequency of all three antigens in the population.

To solve the problem, let us take the total number of people examined (4200) as 100% and calculate in the usual way what percentage are people with genotype $L^M L$.^{M}

$$\frac{1218}{4200} \cdot 100 = 29\%.$$

Hence, the frequency of the $L^M L^M$ genotype is 29%.

The frequency of the other two genotypes can be calculated in the same way. For genotype $L^N L^N$ it is 21%; a $L^M L^N$ - 50%. Expressing the frequencies of the same genotypes in fractions of one, we obtain 0.29; 0.21 and 0.5, respectively.

Other ways of expressing frequency (mainly for rare diseases) are used in population genetics. Suppose that 7 newborns with phenylketonuria out of 69862 newborns are detected in the maternity hospitals of a city. The disease is caused by a recessive gene (a), and the patients are homozygous for this gene (aa). The frequency of the genotype (aa) among the newborns is required.

Recording the frequency using the usual method, we get: $\frac{7}{69862} = 0.0001.$

This method of recording shows that at a given frequency in a population there is one sick child per 10,000 newborns. The same may be written in a more abbreviated form: 1* 10- .^{4}

The composition of the population depends:

1) from previous generations. For example, if in the generation of parents allele (A) was very widespread and allele (a) was rare, then in the generation of descendants genotype (AA) will prevail over genotypes (Aa and aa).

2) from the mutation affecting the generation. For example, if, as a result of mutations in the parental generation, allele (A) mutates into allele (a) with a higher frequency than (a) into (A), then this so-called mutational pressure should influence the ratio of genotypes in the population of descendants by increasing the frequency of allele (a).

3) from natural selection. For example, many mutant genes reduce human viability. Individuals with a mutant gene often die early, leaving no offspring.

4) from the type of marriages. A distinction is made between panmixia, or random marriage, and non-random selection of couples, in which partners with the same or opposite genotype are preferred. Marriage type should be established in relation to a particular heritable trait. For example, in populations, the selection of couples by blood groups is independent of genotype (panmixia), and by height - depending on genotype: people of tall stature are more likely to marry tall people, and stunted people - stunted people.

However, most hereditary traits are not affected by such selection, and panmixia occurs quite widely. Panmixia in human society is also limited by the fact that the populations of some localities and cities consist of relatively isolated groups in which marriages occur predominantly within the group. Such groups are called isolates. In human populations, isolates are due to national, religious, racial, class, and other divisions of society.

The basic regularity allowing to study the genetic structure of populations was established in 1908 independently by the English mathematician G. Hardy and the German physician W. Weinberg. The Hardy-Weinberg law states that in populations under the condition of panmixia and in the absence of mutational and selection pressures, an equilibrium of genotype frequencies is established, which is maintained from generation to generation. From the point of view of population genetic analysis, it is particularly important that the Hardy-Weinberg law establishes a mathematical relationship between gene and genotype frequencies. This dependence is based on a simple mathematical calculation.

Let us observe the behaviour in a population of two alleles (A and a) having arbitrary frequencies (p and q). A cross in such a population can be written as follows: $(pA + qa)\backslash\ x <\$(pA + qa)$. The frequencies of the three possible genotypes obtained in this crossing are expressed by the equation:

(pA + qa)♀ x ♂(pA + qa).

A a AA Aa aa

The letters of the bottom line denote alleles and genotypes, and the corresponding frequencies are located above them in the first line. In its simplest form, the law is described by the formula:

$$p^2AA + 2pqAa + q^2aa = 1.$$

It should be noted that the Hardy-Weinberg law, as well as other genetic regularities based on the Mendelian principle of random combination, is mathematically precisely fulfilled at infinitely large population sizes. In practice, this means that populations with population sizes below a certain minimum value do not fulfil the requirements of the Hardy-Weinberg law. A similar method of calculation can be used for the triallelic system, for example, to study the genetic structure of the population according to the ABO blood group system. In this case, genotypes are determined by alleles I^A , I^B and 1°. Denoting their frequencies by the symbols p, q y, we obtain an expression of the genetic structure of the population:

$$p^2 I^A I^A + q^2 I^B I^B + r^2 I^O I^O + 2\,pr\, I^A I^B + 2qr\, I^A I^O + 2qr\, I^B I^O = 1.$$

This expression quantifies the frequencies of all homozygous and heterozygous genotypes in the ABO blood group system.

Control Questions and Assignments:

1. What methods are used to study human genetics?
2. What is the clinical genealogical method?
3. What questions can be addressed using the clinical genealogical method?
4. What are the main types of inheritance that you know?
5. List the criteria for autosomal dominant type of inheritance and give examples of diseases?
6. List the criteria for autosomal recessive type of inheritance and give examples of diseases?
7. Characterise the differences between X-linked dominant and X-linked recessive types of inheritance?
8. What is the difference between direct and non-direct methods of cytogenetic testing?
9. What biological materials can be used to obtain chromosome

preparations?

10. Name the main methods of chromosome staining?

TEST-7.

1. What causes the disease mucopolysaccharidosis?

а) amino acid metabolism disorders;

б) impaired carbohydrate metabolism;

в) lipid metabolism disorders;

е) chromosomal diseases.

2. Identify the karyotype of Cat Scream Syndrome?

а) 46, XX del(5p);

б) 46, XX, 18q;

(c) 45,HU, t(14q;21q);

е) 46,XX,del(18q).

3. Identify diseases related to autosomal trisomies?

а) Down, Klinefelter;

б) Shereshevsky-Turner, Patau;

(c) Down, Patau, Edwards;

е) Edwards, trisomy X.

4. Which patients have tall stature, eunuchoid physique and gynaecomastia?

а) Klinefelter's syndrome;

б) Marfan syndrome;

(c) Down syndrome;

е) Patau syndrome.

5. In which syndrome are low-set auricles, narrow eye slits, and a short mandible observed?

а) Patau syndrome;

б) Edwards syndrome;

(c) Down syndrome;

е) catcall syndrome.

CHALLENGE-7.

1. In the South American jungle there is an aboriginal population of 127 people (including children). The frequency of blood type M here is 64%. Can we calculate the frequencies of blood group N and MN in this population?

2. Tay-Sachs disease, caused by an autosomal recessive gene, is incurable; people with the disease die in childhood. In one large population, the incidence of affected children is 1:5000.

Will the concentration of the abnormal gene and the incidence of this disease change in the next generation of this population?

3. Congenital hip dislocation is inherited dominantly, with an average gene penetrance of 25%. The incidence is 6:10,000.

Determine the number of homozygous individuals for the recessive gene.

4. Identify the type of inheritance.

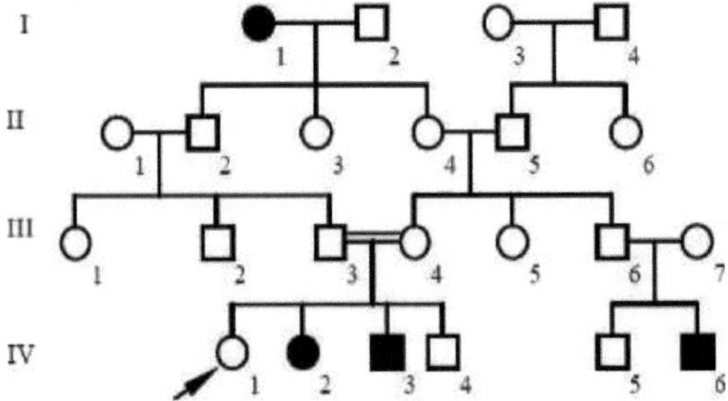

5. The concordance of monozygotic twins in body weight is 80%, and that of dizygotic twins is 30%. What is the ratio of hereditary and environmental factors in the formation of the trait?

CHAPTER VIII

PREVENTION OF HEREDITARY PATHOLOGY

8.1. TYPES OF PREVENTION OF HEREDITARY DISEASES

The profound thought expressed by Leo Tolstoy at the beginning of the novel "Anna Karenina" - "All happy families are similar to each other, every unhappy family is unhappy in its own way" - can be fully applied to families with healthy and sick children. Indeed, every family with a child suffering from a hereditary disease is unhappy in its own way: long-lasting severe illness, early death, mental underdevelopment, etc. Every person wants to have healthy offspring. The deterioration of the environment worldwide and in Uzbekistan in particular aggravates the issue of giving birth to healthy children. All hereditary pathology is determined by genetic "burden", which arises for two reasons.

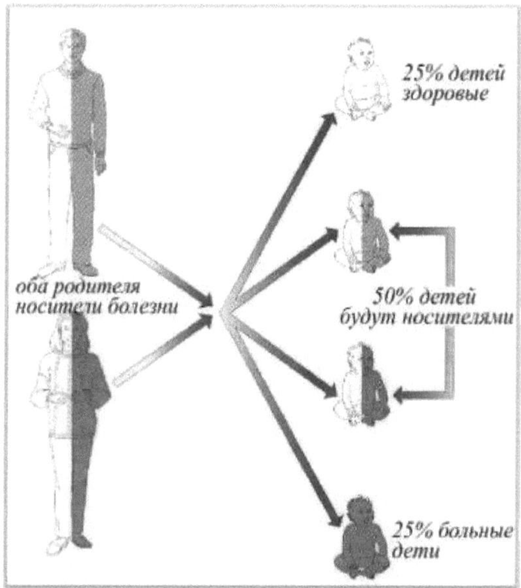

Figure 65. Transmission of a pathological gene to offspring from diseased parents.

1. Segregation - transmission of an abnormal gene to offspring from sick parents or carriers of the abnormal gene (Figure 65).
2. Newly arisen mutation - a change in the hereditary apparatus occurs in the germ cells of healthy parents. As a result, a gamete with a new mutation gives rise to the development of a sick child, although the parents did not have this mutation.

The medical consequences of the "load" of hereditary pathology in humans are manifested by increased mortality, reduced life expectancy, increased number of patients with hereditary diseases, and increased medical care.

Despite the significant advances made in understanding the aetiology and pathogenesis of many hereditary and congenital diseases the achievements in the treatment of these diseases are still not very impressive. This is why the prevention of hereditary diseases must occupy a decisive place in the work of medical personnel and in the organisation of health care.

Prevention is a set of measures aimed at preventing the occurrence and development of hereditary and congenital diseases. There are several types of prevention of hereditary pathology.

Primary prevention is a set of measures aimed at preventing the conception of a sick child. It is realised by planning childbearing and improving the human environment. Planning includes three main positions:

1. Optimal reproductive age, which for women is between 21-35 years (earlier or later pregnancies increase the likelihood of having a child with congenital pathology).
2. Refusal of childbearing in cases of high risk of hereditary and congenital pathology (in the absence of reliable methods of prenatal diagnosis, treatment, adaptation and rehabilitation of patients).
3. Failure to procreate in marriages with blood relatives and between two heterozygous carriers of the pathological gene (see Figure 66).

Secondary prevention is the improvement of the human environment, aimed mainly at preventing newly arising mutations. It is carried out by strict control of the content of mutagens and teratogens in the human environment. The environmental conditions that cause disease are manifold. They include lack of essential nutrients and excessive nutrition, toxic substances and pathogenic microbes, psychogenic and other influences. All these conditions become extreme and pathogenic if they disturb human homeostasis.

Tertiary prevention is carried out through termination of pregnancy in case of high probability of disease in the foetus or diagnosis prenatally. Prenatal diagnosis is carried out with the help of various methods of investigation in the first and second trimesters of pregnancy, i.e. in the periods when it is still possible to terminate the pregnancy in case of pathology detection. Termination can only take place with the woman's consent and within the prescribed time limits. The basis for embryo removal is hereditary disease. Termination of pregnancy is clearly not the best solution, but it is currently the only one suitable for most severe and fatal genetic defects.

The fourth type of prevention of hereditary diseases is aimed at preventing the development of the disease in the born child or its severe manifestations. This form of prevention can be called ***normocopying,*** i.e. the development of a healthy child with a pathological genotype. This prevention of some forms of hereditary pathology may coincide with therapeutic measures in the general medical sense.

Preventing the development of an inherited disease involves a range of treatment measures that can be carried out in utero or after birth. For example, for some inherited diseases such as Rh incompatibility, some acidurias, galactosaemia, intrauterine treatment is possible.

At present, medical and genetic consultations (using prenatal diagnostic methods and neonatal screening) carry out activities aimed at preventing the development of hereditary diseases among the population.

8.2. GENETIC COUNSELLING

Medical and genetic counselling is a type of specialised medical care and can only be carried out by a doctor specialising in medical genetics.

The network of counselling rooms for medical genetics is created on the basis of the health care principles characteristic of the country, taking into account the level of development of medicine in general and the degree of training of medical personnel in clinical genetics. In most foreign countries, counselling is carried out according to a three-stage system:

1. The prognosis of the health of the offspring in the simplest cases is determined by family physicians.
2. More complex cases go to the medical centre's geneticist.
3. Counselling requiring the use of complex genetic methods and calculations is carried out in special genetic counselling centres. Currently, there are about 1,000 institutions around the world that provide medical and genetic counselling in varying amounts. In our country, counselling centres function as an integral part of the existing system of medical care for the population.

The first medical genetics cabinets , which dealt with

In 1971, Academician J.H. Khamidov and Professor A.T. Okilov organised a project on predicting the health of offspring with hereditary pathology at the Tashkent Medical Institute. Many Uzbek scientists have contributed to the development of genetics in Uzbekistan. In recent years, the laboratories of research institutes have been developing problems of medical genetics. The first chairs of medical genetics have been established in the medical faculties of medical institutes. The Ministry of Health of Uzbekistan has issued orders aimed at improving the prevention, diagnosis and treatment of hereditary diseases.

The main aim of genetic counselling is to prevent the birth of a sick child. This applies in particular to severe genetically determined and poorly treatable severe malformations and diseases resulting in physical or mental disability. In accordance with this goal, at the present stage of health care development, medical and genetic counselling should perform the following tasks:

1. Determination of health prognosis for future offspring in families where there was, is or is expected to be a patient with a hereditary pathology;
2. Explaining the meaning of genetic risk to parents in an accessible way and helping them to make decisions about childbearing;
3. Assist physicians in making a diagnosis of an inherited disease when special genetic testing techniques arc rcquired;
4. Dispensary surveillance and identification of a high-risk group among relatives of an individual with an inherited disease;
5. Promotion of medical and genetic knowledge among doctors, nurses and the public.

According to these objectives, the following situations are grounds for referral to counselling:

- delay (disorders) of physical or mental development;
- congenital malformations of internal and external organs;
- specific colour or odour of urine and body odour;
- frequent infectious diseases;
- changes in skin, hair, nails, atrophies;
- skeletal anomalies;
- pathology of the visual organs, cataracts, eye atrophy;
- enlargement of the liver and spleen.

In addition to the signs listed above, it is necessary to suspect hereditary pathology and refer the family to a medical and genetic consultation: in case of similar cases of the disease in relatives; in the presence of spontaneous abortions, stillbirths, children with malformations; in cases of sudden death, parents of women over 35 years of age, men over 45 years of age; in cases of primary infertility.

In the presence of any of these conditions, it is extremely important to consult a geneticist, who will help to exclude or confirm a hereditary disease and determine the necessary recommendations (see Annexes No. 4).

There are ethical issues involved in counselling, such as interference with family privacy or other issues, so health workers, paramedics, must be very careful in interpreting any data.

8.3. PRENATAL DIAGNOSTICS

Prenatal diagnosis is the prenatal detection of congenital or hereditary abnormalities in the foetus. At present, prenatal diagnosis is carried out by means of various research methods in the first and second trimesters of pregnancy, i.e. in the periods when it is still possible to terminate the pregnancy in case of pathology detection. Today it is possible to diagnose almost all chromosomal syndromes and about 100 hereditary diseases in which the biochemical defect has been established reliably.

Prenatal diagnosis uses: non-invasive and invasive methods.

Non-invasive methods of prenatal diagnosis.

Ultrasound (echography) is based on the ability of the ultrasound wave to reflect from the surface of the interface between two media of different densities, which makes it possible to obtain their image on the screen of an electron-beam tube. This study is carried out in the early and later stages of pregnancy, at least twice (12 - 14 weeks and 20 - 21 weeks of pregnancy) when the exact size of the foetus, gestational age, as well as some pathological conditions (undeveloped pregnancy, bubble skid, polyuria, etc.). Ultrasound diagnoses limb malformations, neural tube defects, defects of the anterior abdominal wall, hydro- and microcephaly, heart defects, kidney anomalies.

Biochemical methods include determination of alpha-fetoprotein, chorionic gonadotropin, unbound estradiol levels in the serum of pregnant women. Optimal terms of research 17 - 20 weeks of pregnancy. With the help of biochemical blood tests are diagnosed: multiple pregnancy, intrauterine fetal death, chromosomal diseases of the foetus, etc.

Invasive methods of prenatal diagnosis. Invasive methods include: amniocentesis, chorionbiopsy and cordocentesis, placentocentesis and fetoscopy.

Amniocentesis is performed after a preliminary ultrasound examination, which is used to determine the exact location of the placenta, gestational age and some foetal and uterine malformations. Amniocentesis is a procedure to obtain amniotic fluid (15ml) by puncturing the amniotic sac through the anterior abdominal wall or through the vagina between 16 and 20 weeks of pregnancy (Figure 66). After week 20, the number of "viable" cells decreases significantly. The fluid and cells obtained may be examined cytogenetically or biochemically depending on the suspected fetal pathology. Complications are possible during amniocentesis (premature miscarriage - 1%, infection of the uterine cavity - 0.5%).

Chorionbiopsy (chorionic villus biopsy) is performed at 7-11 weeks' gestation (Figure 67). Visual inspection (ultrasound) is required to take the villi. The villi are taken with biopsy forceps using a plastic catheter. The villous cells grow rapidly at this stage of pregnancy. Chorionic villi cells carry the same genetic information as fetal cells. They can be further analysed using cytogenetic and biochemical methods.

Cordocentesis - blood sampling from the umbilical vein of the foetus is performed between 15 and 22 weeks of pregnancy; some specialists perform this procedure earlier. Culturing leukocytes makes it possible to perform cytogenetic analysis. In addition, biochemical and molecular genctic diagnosis of hereditary diseases without culturing is possible using blood samples.

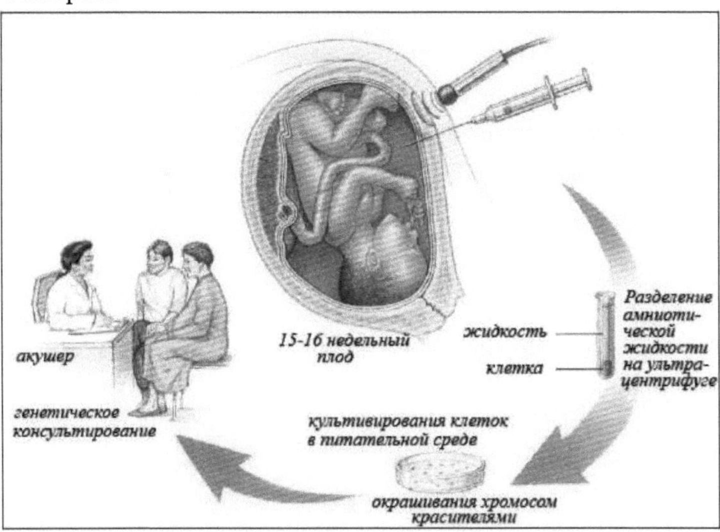

Figure 66. Fetal studies using ultrasound and amniocentesis for prenatal diagnosis.

Fetoscopy is a method of visual observation of the foetus in the uterine cavity through an elastic probe equipped with an optical system. This method is used to diagnose visible congenital malformations, to obtain biopsies of fetal skin and blood from umbilical vessels, which allows the diagnosis of immunodeficiency conditions such as haemoglobinopathies and enzymopathies. It should be noted, however, that the resolving power of fetoscopy is not very high, since only those malformations that are directly in the field of view of the investigator are diagnosed.

Prenatal diagnosis of hereditary diseases and congenital malformations is indicated in the following cases:

- the woman's age is more than 35 years old;
- the presence of structural chromosome rearrangements (especially translocations and inversions) in one of the parents;
- Heterozygous carrier in both parents for autosomal recessive diseases or in the mother alone for X-linked genes;
- The presence of a dominant disease in the parents;
- indication of a history of possible teratogenic effects (radiation, medication and infection during pregnancy, etc.).

Thus, future advances in prenatal diagnosis will be related not only to the improvement of its methodological foundations and the expansion of indications for its performance, but also to public awareness of its ever-increasing possibilities.

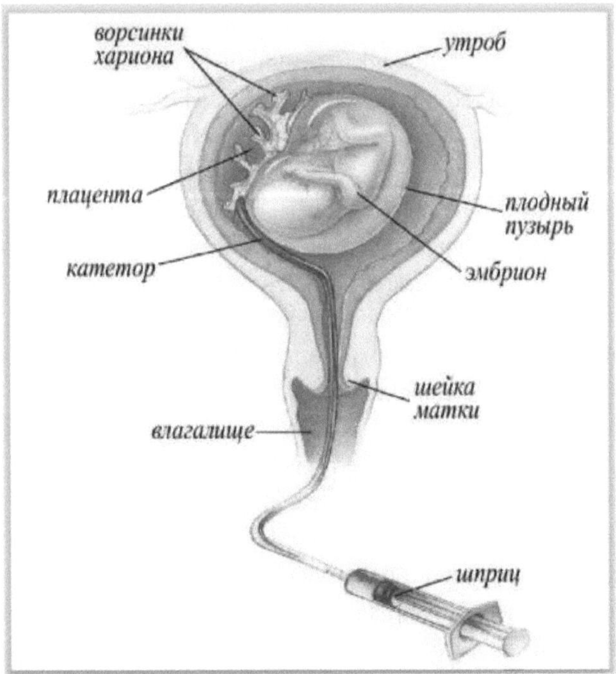

Figure 67. Fetal examination by chorionic villus biopsy.

8.4. HEREDITARY DISEASES

Treatment of patients with hereditary pathologies was until recently considered impossible, but nowadays, after the creation of a number of specific and in many cases highly effective methods of treatment, many hereditary diseases are successfully treated. The success rate of timely treatment is sometimes astonishing. Although today the fight against hereditary pathology is a matter of specialised scientific institutions, it is thought that the time is not far off when patients after diagnosis and the beginning of pathogenetic treatment will come under the supervision of doctors of ordinary clinics and polyclinics. This requires the practical doctor and nursing staff to know the basic methods of treatment of hereditary pathology, both existing and under development (see Appendix 5).

Several treatments are used in the treatment of hereditary diseases and diseases with hereditary predisposition:

1. Substitution therapy.
2. Vitamin therapy.
3. Nutritional therapy.

4. Surgical treatment, etc.

Replacement therapy. The meaning of replacement therapy for inherited metabolic errors is simple: the introduction of missing or insufficient biochemical substrates into the body. A classic example of replacement therapy is the treatment of diabetes mellitus. The use of insulin has dramatically reduced not only mortality from this disease, but also the disability of patients.

Substitution therapy is also successfully used in other endocrine diseases - iodine and thyroidine preparations for hereditary defects in the synthesis of thyroid hormones, well known to clinicians as androgenital syndrome. The treatment of haemophilia by transfusion of donor blood and administration of antihaemophilic globulin is based on the same principle. The treatment of Parkinson's disease has proved to be highly effective. The administration of the necessary amino acids to patients significantly alleviates the symptoms of the disease and especially reduces muscle rigidity.

However, replacement therapy of hereditary metabolic diseases is hindered by the fact that many enzyme abnormalities are localised in cells of the central nervous system, liver, etc. Delivery to these target organs of certain enzyme substrates is difficult, since their introduction into the body develops corresponding immunopathological reactions. As a result, inactivation or complete destruction of the enzyme occurs. Currently, new methods are being developed to prevent this phenomenon.

Vitamin therapy. This is the treatment of certain hereditary metabolic diseases by the administration of vitamins, very similar to replacement therapy. However, in replacement therapy, normal doses of biochemical substrates are administered, whereas in vitamin therapy, doses ten times larger are administered. For example, the disease "urine with the smell of maple syrup" is inherited by the autosomal recessive type. In this disease isovalerian acid and other metabolic products of keto acids are excreted from the body in large quantities, which gives the urine a specific odour. Symptomatology consists of muscular rigidity, seizure syndrome and nervous system disorders. One form of the disease is successfully treated with excessive doses of vitamin B_1 from the first days of the child's life. The results of early treatment with high doses of vitamin B1 are very encouraging.

Diet therapy (therapeutic nutrition). In many hereditary metabolic diseases is the only pathogenetic and very successful method of treatment, and in some cases a method of prevention. The latter fact is all the more important because only a few hereditary metabolic disorders (e.g., intestinal lactose deficiency) develop in adults. Usually the disease manifests itself either in the first hours (cystic fibrosis, galactosemia) or in the first weeks (phenylketonuria) of a child's life and leads more or less quickly to unfortunate consequences, up to death.

The simplicity of the basic therapeutic measure - the elimination of a certain factor from the diet - remains extremely tempting. However, although in no other disease does nutritional therapy stand alone as an effective treatment method, it requires strict adherence to a number of conditions and a clear understanding of the complexity of obtaining the desired result.

Surgical treatment. This type of treatment occupies a significant place in the care of patients with hereditary pathology. Often the need for surgical correction arises immediately after birth (oesophageal stenosis and atresia, anus atresia, etc.).

Transplantation of organs and tissues as a method of treatment of hereditary diseases is currently widely used in medical practice.

Plastic surgery is widely used in the treatment of various developmental anomalies in children and adults.

The considered methods of treatment of hereditary diseases by virtue of the established etiology or pathogenetic links can be considered specific. However, for the absolute majority of hereditary pathologies, we do not yet have methods of specific therapy. This applies, for example, to chromosomal syndromes, although their etiological factors are well known, or to such diseases with hereditary predisposition as atherosclerosis and hypertension, although some mechanisms of development of these diseases are more or less studied.

Treatment of both turns out to be symptomatic rather than specific. The fatality of hereditary diseases exists only as long as their causes and pathogenesis are not understood.

8.5. PHARMOCOGENETICS

It is well known from medical practice that when treated with the same drug, some patients have hypersensitivity to it. Reasons in the reaction to drugs can be not only the physiological state of the body, age, sex, but also genetic features. The role of heredity in the body's reactions to drugs is studied by a special section of genetics - *pharmocogenetics.* One of the tasks of pharmocogenetics is to study the causes of atypical reactions to drugs, in particular, to identify disorders of enzymatic mechanisms of metabolism, their conditioning by genetic factors and the distribution of these factors in the population.

It is also necessary to find out whether genetic factors are involved in the diversity of reactions of the organism to drugs. It has been established that the uniqueness of the organism's genotype may cause differences between individuals in the nature and rate of drug metabolism. This is manifested not by clinical pathology, but by a peculiar therapeutic effect and severity of side effects.

A doctor or nurse may encounter this problem many times in their practice. For example, an individual's hypersensitivity to a medicine, as happens in cases of overdose, even though the patient is prescribed a dose appropriate for his or her age and sex. The presence of complete tolerance in the patient to the drug, even though the dose is increased. The development of paradoxical reactions to the drug, including very different types of complications than would be expected based on the mechanisms of action of the drug.

Let's look at some examples:

1. In the early 1950s, a new effective drug, isoniazid, began to be used for the treatment of tuberculosis. Toxic effects were observed in some patients when using standard doses. The reason for this phenomenon turned out to be that toxic effects of isoniazid are hereditary in nature. There is a family accumulation of such cases of "overdose" from the usual doses and the excretion of isoniazid from the body in such patients is slow. This depends on the enzyme that removes isoniazid from the body (N-acetyltransferase). If the enzyme is normal, then in such individuals the drug is eliminated from the body within 2 h, if the enzyme is abnormal, then the drug is eliminated from the body slowly (after 6 h). If the drug is taken into the body regularly, its reduced excretion leads to cumulation (accumulation) of the drug in the body and its accumulation to a toxic dose.
2. In some families, in addition to healthy individuals, there are family members who are resistant to anticoagulant drugs. This is due to a genetically determined mutant form of vitamin K metabolism involved in blood coagulation. In some patients with evident signs of rickets, the use of vitamin D in standard doses does not lead to a therapeutic effect. This hereditary disease is called *vitamin D-resistant rickets or hypophosphatemia.* The key link in the disease is a decrease in phosphate reabsorption in the renal tubules.

3. We have considered some of the most studied hereditary metabolic defects that are detected only when the organism comes into contact with the corresponding drug. However, a large group of inherited diseases are accompanied by atypical reactions to drugs. One such inherited metabolic defect is the pronounced resistance of some individuals to the action of hydrocyanic acid and its salts. For example, they can administer a dose of potassium cyanide forty times more lethal without serious consequences.

In history, there is a case that has received almost mystical interpretation. One of the close associates of Emperor Nicholas II, Grigory Rasputin, tried to poison with potassium cyanide in a dose known to exceed lethal. However, after eating poisoned food Rasputin had no signs of poisoning. In terms of pharmocogenetics, this unique case of resistance to the strongest poison can be explained by the fact that Rasputin was a mutant on the gene determining variants of haemoglobin.

4. Gout is inherited in an autosomal dominant type with incomplete penetrance and is manifested by accelerated synthesis of uric acid with a simultaneous decrease in its excretion by the kidneys. Accumulation of urates in tissues leads to inflammatory reactions in joints and formation of kidney stones.

Elevated blood sugar (diabetes mellitus), is often inherited as an autosomal recessive trait. The symptomatology of this disease is well known. However, there are a variety of forms of diabetes mellitus. For example, insulin dependent and insulin independent.

In case of hereditarily determined but latent tendency to gout and diabetes, some diuretics (drugs: chlorthiazite, furosemide) can either provoke the first clinical signs of the diseases or sharply intensify their development.

Thus, pharmacogenetic studies have made it possible to describe a number of metabolic defects affecting the body's sensitivity to drugs. The need to diagnose hereditary anomalies of drug metabolism is more than obvious, as this will avoid many complications or cases of ineffective treatment. Based on knowledge of the human genome, high-resolution methods have now been developed to recognise mutations in genes that enable drug metabolism. Consequently, drug treatment strategies in the new millennium will include genotyping patients before initiating therapy.

Control Questions and Assignments:

1. Give a definition of the term prevention.
2. What types of prevention do you know?
3. What is medical genetic counselling?
4. What are the objectives of medical and genetic counselling?

5. List the principles of referral to medical and genetic counselling.
6. List the signs on the basis of which a hereditary pathology can be suspected.
7. What is prenatal diagnosis?
8. State the indications for prenatal diagnosis.
9. List non-invasive and invasive diagnostic methods.
10. What treatments for hereditary diseases do you know?

TEST-8.

1. Define the karyotype of Down syndrome?
(a)46,XX+21;
b) 47,XU+21;
(c) 47,HU+18;
e) 47, XX+13.
2. In which syndrome are low-set auricles, narrow eye slits, and a short mandible observed?
a) Patau syndrome;
б) Edwards syndrome;
в) Down syndrome;
e) catcall syndrome.
3. What type of inheritance is Daltonism?
a) autosomal dominant;
б) autosomal recessive;
в) X-linked dominant;
e) X-linked recessive.
4. Where are the allelic genes located?
a) in different (non-homologous) chromosomes;
б) in one chromosome;
(c) In identical loci of homologous chromosomes;
e) in different loci of non-homologous chromosomes.
5. Select the most complete definition of analytical crossbreeding.
a) crossbreeding to clarify genotype and phenotype;
б) crossing an organism with a dominant phenotype and unknown genotype with an organism that has a recessive phenotype;
(c) Crossbreeding of phenotypically similar organisms;
e) crossbreeding by an unknown genotypic organism.

CHALLENGE-8:

1. identify the type of inheritance.

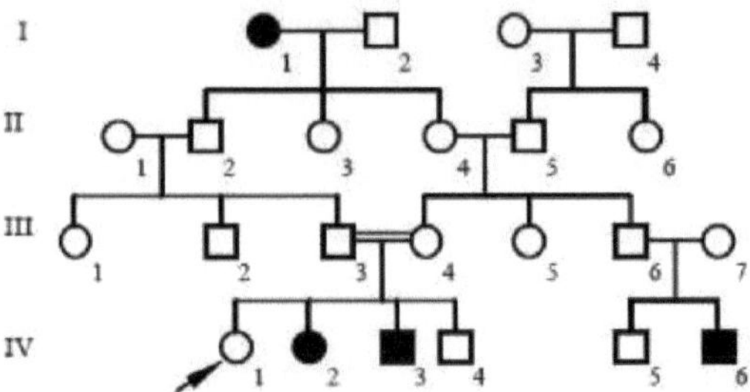

2. Identify the type of inheritance.

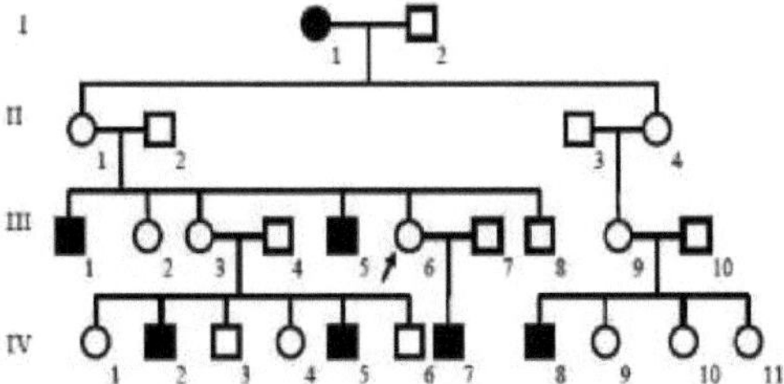

3. Identify the type of inheritance.

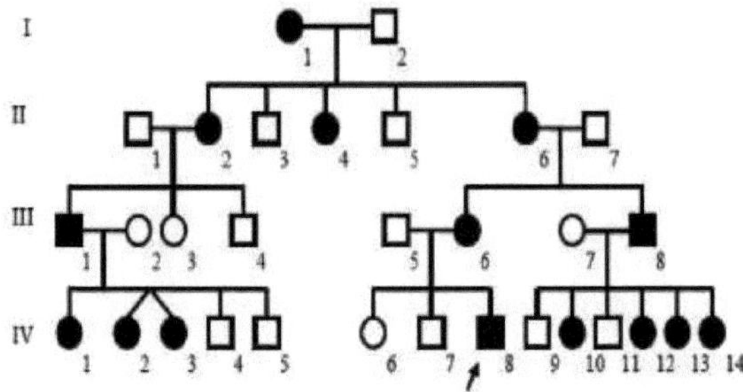

4. A man and his son have haemophilia. The man's wife is pregnant. Fearing that her son would be born haemophiliac, she went to a medical genetic clinic to determine the sex of the foetus and to terminate the pregnancy if it turned out that the foetus was male. After talking to her, the doctors recommended that she terminate the pregnancy immediately without amniocentesis. Is this recommendation correct?

5. Which of the following symptoms are diagnostic signs of Marfan syndrome:

a) mental retardation, enlargement of the liver and spleen, generalised dystrophy, cataracts;

б) microcephaly, microphthalmia, bilateral cleft lip and palate, syndactyly

of the toes, heart septal defects, mental retardation;
в) subluxation of the lens, heart defects, tall stature, long thin fingers, funnel-shaped depression of the sternum;
г) blue sclerae, congenital deafness, brittle bones;
д) flat face, low sloping forehead, light spots on the iris, thick tongue protruding from the mouth, deformed low-set auricles, atrial septal defect, mental retardation?

Appendix 1.

Human chromosome maps

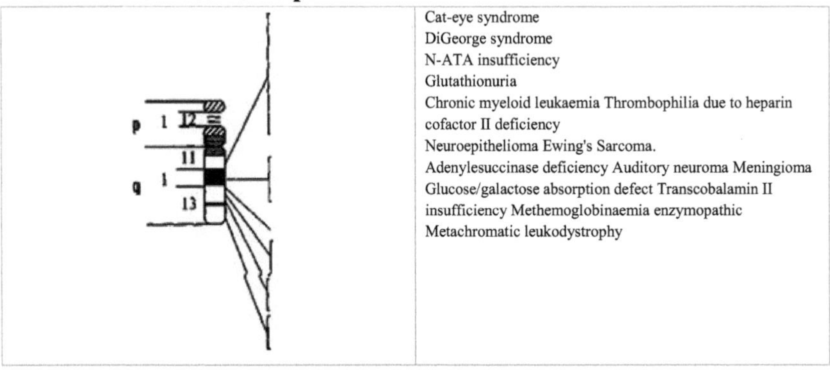

Map of the 22nd human chromosome

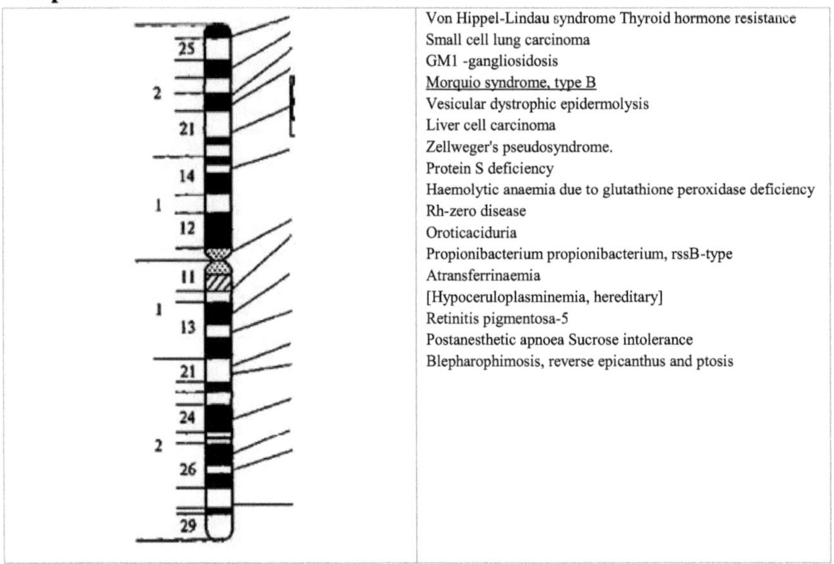

Map of human chromosome 3

Clinical classification of hereditary diseases

Diagnostic index of syndromes	№	Diseases	Clinical manifestation
(a) Diseases caused by metabolic disorders.	1.	Albinism.	It's based on an inherited defect. of melanin metabolism , resulting in reduced or absent pigment in the skin, mucous membranes hair, eyes. Three clinical forms are distinguished: ocular (inherited recessively X-linked), cutaneous, ocular cutaneous (inherited autosomal recessively).
	2.	Galactosemia.	Symptoms may appear as soon as the baby starts getting milk : vomiting, decreased weight loss , jaundice, progressive hepatomegaly, ascites, dyspepsia, cataracts, dementia. In the severe form, death occurs. In the mild form, the symptoms are less severe.
	3.	Glycogenosis.	Hereditary group enzymopathies characterised by excessive accumulation of glycogen in the glycogen different organs and tissues due to disruption of its breakdown and synthesis processes. Eleven types have been studied. Specific treatment of diseases of this group has not been developed.
	4.	Marfan syndrome.	See topic 7.1.1.
	5.	Progeria.	Manifested from birth or early in life by growth retardation and underweight, and by
) Diseases of the musculoskeletal system.	6. 1. 2.	Atopias (Allergic diseases). Achard's syndrome. Congenital dislocations	skin changes. The skin is thin, shiny, dry (reduced sweating), tightly stretched. On the arms and legs the skin is loose, wrinkled. In

		of the hip.	the lower abdomen and upper thigh, the skin is thickened, rough, reminiscent of scleroderma . Veins are visible due to lack of subcutaneous fat layer. Normal build, large head, micrognathia, beak-shaped nose , ears. are spurred. Life expectancy from 7 to 27 years. Clinical manifestations , conditioned perverted reaction of the organism to certain environmental stimuli: bronchial asthma, hay fever , vasomotor rhinitis , exudative diathesis, etc. Familial spread has long been noted, but the pathogenesis and genetic mechanisms have not been established. It's manifesting itself arachnodactyly, oblique. small lower jaw, limited mobility. the joints of the arms and legs. The broad skull, pronounced brachycephaly and small jaw distinguish this syndrome from Marfan's disease. There are three degrees of deformity in terms of severity: dysplasia, subluxation and dislocation of the hip. Dysplasia is the mildest degree of the disease manifested by an offence tissue ossification In subluxations, the head of the femur is partially outside the hip socket. Hip dislocation is the most severe degree, in which the

			femoral head is out of the
			hollows. Genetically. deterministic forms are inherited by autosomal dominance with a high degree of The predominance of left-sided joint involvement is predominant in females.
	3.	Gout.	It's characterised by joint pain, joint changes . configuration, limitation mobility. Small joints are more often affected. There are no inflammatory changes in the joints. Disease progresses , leading to ankylosis, renal stone attacks are common. of the disease. Serum levels of uric acid are elevated, which salts are deposited in the joints.
c)Diseases of the endocrine system.	1.	Bardet-Biedl or Lawrence-Moon syndrome.	The main clinical signs are obesity, degeneration. retinal, genital. hypoplasia, polydactyly, mental retardation. In addition to the main features, acrocephaly, syndactyly, dwarfism or gigantism, anal atresia, deafness, etc. may be present. In adult patients, there are signs of dysfunctional deficiency of the pituitary gland. Women underdevelopment of the mammary glands, gynaecomastia in men, etc.
	2.	Klinefelter's syndrome.	See topic 5.8.
	3.	Shereshevsky-Turner syndrome.	See topic 5.8.
	4.	Pendred's syndrome	It's characterised by an enlarged

		(Goiter with deafness).	thyroid gland , as in usually euthyroid. Deafness or hearing loss with decreased perception of high tones is often combined with the following
d) Heart and vascular diseases.	1.	Holt-Orumm syndrome.	vestibular disorders. The syndrome is based on impaired tyrosine iodination. See topic 7.1.1.
	2.	Wolff-Hirschhorn syndrome.	It's characterised by severe hypotrophy, retardation. mental and physical development; microcephaly, hypertelorism, small, low ears, cleft lip and palate, seizures. Asymmetry of the skull and brain defects have been described in some patients , hemangiomas on the eyebrows, epicanthus, antimongoloid eyes, micrognathia. Dysplasia. joints and congenital heart defects. The disease is caused by a deletion of the short arm of the 4th chromosome.
	3.	Mucopolysaccharidoses.	See topic 5.4.2.
	4.	Haemophilia.	See Theme 3.2 Characterised by spontaneousi post-traumatic haemorrhages, localised most often in the large joints of the limbs with subsequent development ankyloses and deformities of the joints. Sometimes haemorrhages occur gastrointestinally. intestinal tract, kidneys, nasal cavity.
	5.	Thalassaemia (Cooley's disease).	There are three types: small, large (Cooley's anaemia) and intermediate thalassaemia . Familial hereditary haemolytic anaemia

			is common in populations along the Mediterranean coast. Thalassaemia syndrome caused by a hereditary deterministic decrease in globin synthesis. Accordingly, a - T and p-T are distinguished.
			The first form is much less common, but in a - T the synthesis of all three types of haemoglobin is impaired , (HbA, HbF and HbA2). In p-T, only HbA synthesis is impaired. See topic 3.2.
e) Diseases of the eyes, skin, nails, hair and mucous membranes.	1.	Ayres Disease.	It manifests as inflammation of the red lip area, usually the lower lip. Cheilitnositis actinic in nature. It is based on an increased sensitivity to sunlight. Type of inheritance autosomal dominant.
	2.	Albinism.	See topic 5.4.1.
	3.	Hypotrichosis (Wean's Syndrome).	It's characterised by a congenital lack of pubescent hair, late development of bristly and long hair and early hair loss up to complete alopetition.
	4.	Hypertrichosis.	Excessive hair growth on all parts of the body except palms, soles and mucous membranes. Hypertrichosis is noted from birth and becomes more severe later in life, and may diminish by puberty.
	5.	Vitiligo.	Manifested by the formation round and hammered depigmented spots , The disease is more common in women between 8 months and 20 years of age. Women aged 8 months to 20 years are more often affected. The pathogenesis of vitiligo is poorly understood.

(e) Diseases of the neuromuscular system.	1.	Leukodystrophy.	Hereditary group diseases of the nervous system characterised by progressive decay white matter of brain tissue due to enzyme defects.
			involved in lipid catabolism and myelin synthesis.
	2.	Schizophrenia (Blyler's disease). Ptosis. Albinism.	It's manifested by increasing changes in the personality in the form of disruption of its unity, loss of connection with reality , peculiar offences thinking. By the nature of the course there are several variants: neurosis-like, affective, hallucinatory , delusional, catatonic. The role of hereditary factors is evident. It is generally believed that schizophrenia is determined by a number of factors, some of which are inherited monogenically, others polygenically. Ptosis is most often caused by underdevelopment or absence of the muscle that raises the upper eyelid, less often it is associated with aplasia of the lateral paired nuclei of the oculomotor nerve or its fibres. Ptosis can be bilateral and bilateral, full and incomplete. Incomplete In bilateral ptosis, the patient's head is tilted back (stargazer's pose), the skin folds on the forehead are pronounced.
	3.		
g) Diseases of the ear, throat, nose and facial anomalies.	1.		See topic 5.4.1.
	2.	Catcall syndrome or (Lejeune's syndrome).	See topic 5.7.

karyotype recording examples

PHENOTYPE	CARIOTYPE
A normal man	46, HU.
A normal woman.	46,XX
Male with Down syndrome, simple trisomy 21	47, HU, +21
A normal male Robertson translocation carrier. (e.g. father of a child with a translocation form of Down syndrome)	45, HU, t(14q; 21q)
A girl with Patau syndrome, simple trisomy 13.	47, XX,+13
A boy with Edwards syndrome, simple trisomy 18.	47,KHU,+18.
A girl with "cat cry" syndrome (short arm deletion chromosome 5)	46, XX, 5p or 46, XX del(5p)
A girl with malformations (long arm deletion chromosome 18)	46, XX, 18q or 46, XX, del (18q)
A man with chronic myeloleukaemia	46, XU, t(9q34; 22qll)*
Turner syndrome (monosomy of the X chromosome).	45,X
Normal female (X-chromosome number mosaicism)	46, XX/47, XXX
A man with Klinefelter's syndrome	47 XXU.
Normal girl (pericentric inversion of chromosome 7)	46, XX, inv(7) (p14q25)
A normal male with polysemy U	47, HUU.
Girl with genital malformation (isochromosome on the long arm of the X chromosome)	46, X, i(Xq)

* A small marker chromosome 22, the so-called "Philadelphia chromosome", labelled (Ph), is found in the karyotype.

The rules for recording karyotypes:

1. The total number of chromosomes (e.g. 45, 46, 47, etc.) is indicated at the beginning;
2. Then the composition of the sex chromosomes (e.g., XX, XU, XO, XXU, etc.);
3. An added autosome is indicated by a (+) sign or the loss of an entire chromosome is indicated by a (-) sign, e.g. 21+, 21-;
4. The short shoulder is denoted by the Latin letters "p", the long shoulder by "q";
5. The translocation is denoted by the letter "1" with decoding in brackets (e.g., 1(14+21)- carrier of a balanced translocation 14/21: 1(14+21)- carrier of balanced translocation 14/21);
6. Mosaicism is indicated by a fraction sign (e.g.: 45,X/46,XX - mosaicism in Shereshevsky-Terner syndrome).

Brief characterisation of some monogenic hereditary diseases

Disease	Minimum diagnostic criterion	Inheritance type	The most frequent requests
Aarski syndrome	Hypertelorism, brachydactyly, cutaneous. syndactyly, short stature, floppy scrotum.	BP or X-z. P	Endocrinologist
Aglossia-adactyly	Microgenia, micro- or	AD	Surgeon

syndrome (Hanhart syndrome)	aglossia, reduction. limb defects		
Adrenogenital syndrome	Progressive virilisation, dual genitalia, accelerated somatic development	AP	Endocrinologist
Acrocephalosin-dactylia.	Acrocephaly, varying degrees of syndactyly	AD	Neurosurgeon, surgeon
Albinism ocular-cutaneous tyrosinazonegative-albinism	Depigmentation of skin, hair, eyes, photophobia, nystagmus	AP	Ophthalmologist
Alport syndrome (hereditary nephritis with deafness)	Hearing loss, haematuria and proteinuria	AD, X- cc. P	Neurologist, otolaryngologist
Ataxia-telangiectasia (Luibar syndrome)	Ataxia, telangiectasia, recurrent upper respiratory infections pathways, decreased IgA levels	AP	Neurologist
Bardet-Biedl syndrome	Obesity, hypogonadism, mental retardation, polydactyly	AP	Endocrinologist, neuropsychologist, ophthalmologist
Beckwith-Wiedemann syndrome	Omphalocele, macroglossia, macrosomia	AD	Surgeon
Williams syndrome (elf-face syndrome).	Unusual face , supravalvular aortic stenosis, mental retardation , hypercalcaemia	AD	Psychoneurologist, cardiac surgeon.
Tay-Sachs' amaurotic idiocy.	Psychomotor retardation, muscular. hypotension, blindness, early death.	AP	Paediatric neurologist
Hymophilia A	Haemorrhages, haemarthroses, factor VIII deficiency	H-Sc. P	Haematologist
disease	**Minimum Diagnostic Criterion**	**Inheritance type**	**The most frequent requests**
Marfan syndrome	High growth , arachnodactyly, subluxation of the lens , aortic aneurysm	AD	Cardiac surgeon ophthalmologist
Larsen syndrome	Multiple congenital	ADi AR	Orthopaedist

	dislocations , unusual face, skeletal anomalies.		
Duchenne muscular dystrophy	Muscle weakness , pseudohypertrophy of the calf muscles, progressive course	H-Sc. P	Neurologist
Neurofibromatosis (Recklin-Gausen disease).	pigment spots , multiple neurofibromas, optic nerve glioma	AD	Neurologist, dermatologist
Osteogenesis imperfecta	Increased fragility bones, blue sclerae, otosclerosis.	ADi AR	Surgeon, otolaryngologist
Russell-Silver syndrome	Stunted, peculiar face , skeletal asymmetry, sexual dysfunction. developments	AD	Endocrinologist
Rubinstein-Teiby syndrome	progressive mental retardation , broad nail phalanges of the first fingers and toes, characteristic face	AD	Psychoneurologist
Usher syndrome	Congenital sensorineural deafness, retinitis pigmentosa	AP	Surdologist, otolaryngologist, ophthalmologist

Note: AD - autosomal dominant type of inheritance;

AR is an autosomal recessive type of inheritance;

X- chromosome. P - recessive linked to the X chromosome.

Characteristics of inherited diseases detected through newborn screening

Disease	Defect (most frequent)	Clinical Manifestation	Correction
Phenylketonuria	Phenylalene ninhydroxylase deficiency.	Constipation, eczematous skin lesions, psychomotor retardation, microcephaly, mental retardation	Restriction of phenylalanine-containing foods in the child's diet
Galactosemia	Galactose -1 phosphaturidyltrans-ferase deficiency	Physical and mental retardation, vomiting, liver damage, cataracts, mental retardation, early death	A diet completely devoid of galactose

Congenital hypothyroidism	Disorder of thyroid hormone biosynthesis	Dry skin, constipation, neurological disorders, goitre, myxedema, dementia	Thyroid hormone replacement therapy
Adrenogenital syndrome	Insufficiency 21-hydroxylases	There are several clinical variants. In the frequent virile form there is precocious puberty in boys and muscularisation in girls External genitalia. With a salt-lowering diet, collapse.	Assignment glucocorticosteroid drugs, mineralocorticoids
Cystic fibrosis	Abnormality of a protein that is a transmembrane regulator of chloride conductance in cells	Cough, recurrent bronchitis , sinusitis, pneumonia, profuse stool , pancreatic pathology	Mucolytics, pacreatic enzymes, antibiotic therapy respiratory exercise programme

GLOSSARY OF GENETIC TERMS

Chromosomal aberration (or chromosomal abnormality): 1) a generalised name for any of the types of chromosomal mutations - deletions, translocations, inversions, duplications; 2) genomic mutations (aneuploidies, trisomies, etc.).

Agenesia (aplasia) is the complete congenital absence of an organ or part of an organ.

Acrocephaly (oxycephaly) is an abnormally high or conical shape of the skull.

An allele is one of two, or more, alternative forms of a gene, each characterised by a unique nucleotide sequence.

Alopecia (baldness, baldness) is permanent or temporary, complete or partial hair loss.

Alpha-fetoprotein (AFP) is an embryonic protein found in the blood of the foetus of a newborn, pregnant woman, and in amniotic fluid.

Amniocentesis is a puncture of the amniotic sac to obtain amniotic fluid.

Anaphase is the phase of mitotic and meiotic division of the nucleus.

Aneuploidy is **an** altered set of chromosomes in which one or more chromosomes from the normal set are either missing or represented by extra copies.

Anotia is aplasia of the auricles.

Anophthalmia is the absence of one or both eyeballs.

Anticodon is a group of three bases complementary to the codon in iRNA. It occupies a fixed position in the tRNA molecule.

Antimongoloid eye section - the external corners of the eye slits are lowered.

Arachnodactyly - unusually long and thin fingers.

Atresia is the complete absence of a canal or natural opening.

An aut**osome** is any non-sex chromosome. Humans have 22 pairs of autosomes.

Autosomal dominant inheritance **- a** type of inheritance in which a single mutant allele localised in an autosome is sufficient for a disease (or trait) to manifest.

Chorion biopsy - a procedure performed at 7-11 weeks of pregnancy to obtain cells for prenatal diagnosis. **Blepharophimosis** - horizontal shortening of the eyelids, i.e. narrowing of the eye slits.

Brachydactyly is a shortening of the fingers.

Brachycephaly is an increase in the transverse size of the head with a relative decrease in the longitudinal size.

Vitiligo is focal depigmentation.

Congenital diseases - diseases present at birth.

A **gamete** is a mature sex cell.

Haemangiomas (angiomas) are congenital benign vascular neoplasms.

Hemizygosity is the state of an organism in which some gene is represented in a single chromosome.

A gene is a sequence of nucleotides in DNA that determines a specific function in an organism or ensures transcription of another gene.

Genetic engineering is a set of techniques, methods and technologies for obtaining recombinant RNA and DNA, isolation of genes from organisms (cells), manipulation of genes and their introduction into other organisms.

Gene therapy is the introduction of genetic material (DNA or RNA) into a cell whose function it changes (or the function of an organism).

Genome - the total genetic information contained in the genes of an organism, or the genetic makeup of a cell. The term "genome" is sometimes used to refer to the haploid set of chromosomes.

Genotype: 1) all the genetic information of an organism;
2) genetic characterisation of an organism at one or more loci under study.

The gene pool is the set of genes of a species or population.

Heterozygote - a cell (or organism) containing two different alleles at a locus of homologous chromosomes.

A heterozygous organism is an organism that has two different forms of a given gene (different alleles) in homologous chromosomes.

Heterochromatin is a region of a chromosome (sometimes an entire chromosome) that has a dense compact structure in interphase and is not transcribed into RNA.

Iris heterochromia is an uneven colouration of different parts of the iris.

Hybrid - an individual resulting from the crossing of genetically different parental forms.

In situ hybridisation **is** hybridisation between denatured cellular DNA on a slide and single-stranded RNA or DNA labelled with radioactive isotopes or immunofluorescent compounds.

Hyperhidrosis - increased sweating as a manifestation of excessive sweat gland function.

Hypertelorism - increased distance between the inner edges of the eye sockets.

Nipple hypertelorism is an increased distance between the nipples.

Hypertrichosis is the presence of coarse, long, pigmented hair in places where downy hair would normally be.

Hypospadias is a lower urethral cleft with displacement of the external opening of the urethral valve.

Hypotelorism - reduced distance between the inner edges of the eye sockets.

Hirsutism is excessive male-type hair loss in girls.

Golandric inheritance **is** inheritance linked to the U chromosome.

Blue sclerae (blue) - blue colouring of the sclerae is due to the translucency of the vasculature through the thinning sclera.

Homozygote - a cell (or organism) containing two identical alleles at a particular locus of homologous chromosomes.

A homozygous organism is an organism that has two identical copies of a given gene in homologous chromosomes.

Homologous chromosomes are chromosomes that are identical in terms of the set of genes that make up them.

Linkage group - all genes localised in one chromosome.

Gene fingerprinting - detecting variations in the number and length of DNA tandem repeats.

Deletion: 1) a type of chromosomal mutation in which a section of a chromosome is lost; 2) a type of gene mutation in which a section of a DNA molecule is dropped.

Distichiasis is a double row of eyelashes.

Dolichocephaly - predominance of longitudinal head dimensions over transverse head dimensions.

Dominant - a trait or corresponding allele that is expressed in heterozygotes.

Gene drift is a change in gene frequencies in a series of generations due to random events resulting from limited sampling of gametes.

Duplication: 1) a type of chromosomal mutation in which a section of a chromosome is doubled; 2) a type of gene mutation in which a section of DNA is doubled.

Genetic probe - a short piece of DNA or RNA of known structure or function labelled with some radioactive or fluorescent compound.

Variability - differences between individuals belonging to the same species.

An isochromosome is an aberrant monocentric chromosome with two genetically identical arms.

Genomic (gene or chromosomal) **imprinting** is a mechanism by which the activity of homologous genes (or sections of chromosomes) in an individual differs depending on the parental sex.

Inbreeding is the mating of related individuals.

Inbred marriages **are** marriages between blood relatives of the 2nd or further degree of consanguinity.

Inversion: 1) a type of chromosomal mutation in which the sequence of genes in a section of chromosomes is reversed; 2) a type of gene mutation in which the sequence of bases in a particular section of DNA is reversed.

Insertion is a type of gene mutation in which there is an insertion of a piece of DNA into the gene structure.

Interphase is the period of a cell's life cycle between the end of one mitosis and the beginning of the next.

Intron - a segment of DNA in a gene that does not contain information about the structure of the protein product of the gene.

Ichthyosis - "scaly" skin, the presence of dense greyish scales on the skin resembling fish scales.

Karyotype is the chromosome set of a cell or organism.

Gene cloning is the production of millions of identical copies of a particular section of DNA using microorganisms for this purpose.

Clinodactyly is a lateral or medial curvature of the finger.

Codominant alleles are alleles that are each expressed in heterozygote (e.g., blood type AB).

A codon is a word (figuratively) in the language of the genetic code. In essence, a codon is three adjacent bases that ensure the inclusion of one amino acid residue in a polypeptide chain, or signal the start or end of transcription.

Colinearity - correspondence of the sequence of amino acids in a polypeptide chain to the order of codons encoding it in iRNA.

A compound is an organism that is heterozygous for two mutant alleles of the same locus.

A **coloboma** is the absence or usually a sectoral defect of a structure, most commonly of the eye, such as a coloboma of the iris, coloboma of the lens.

Concordance is the identity of a trait in twins.

Cordocentesis is a procedure to draw blood from the umbilical vein of the fetus.

Inbreeding coefficient is the probability that one individual has two alleles at a given locus from the same ancestor.

Crossingover - the process of exchanging genes or homologous parts of homologous chromosomes during meiosis, provides new combinations of genes.

Lethal - a mutation that causes the death of a cell or individual before reaching reproductive age.

Lysosomal diseases are a group of inherited diseases characterised by inherited deficient production of lysosomal enzymes.

Lipomas are subcutaneous tumour masses.

Liposomes are spherical particles artificially derived from a bimolecular layer of lipids.

A **locus** is a place on a chromosome occupied by a gene.

Macroglossia is an enlarged tongue.

Macrosomia (gigantism) - excessively enlarged body size, when height and weight indicators significantly exceed the age and sex norms.

Macrostomia - an excessively wide mouth slit.

Macrotia - enlarged auricles.

Macrocephaly - increased size of the skull.

A marker is an allele (or trait) whose inheritance is traceable in the offspring.

Meiosis - two consecutive (1st and 2nd) divisions of the nucleus of a germ (sex) cell at one replication cycle, resulting in haploid cells.

Mendelisation - inheritance of a certain trait (disease) in accordance with H. Mendel's laws.

Metaphase is the stage of mitosis during which the spiralised chromosomes are arranged in the equatorial plane of the cell.

Microgenia - small size of the mandible.

Micrognathia - small size of the upper jaw.

Microcephaly is the small size of the brain and cerebral skull.

Microphthalmia - small size of the eyeball.

Mixoplasm is the state of intracellular matter after fusion of the contents of the nucleus (karyoplasm) and cytoplasm.

Missense mutations are gene mutations that change the meaning of a codon and, consequently, lead to the replacement of one amino acid with another that cannot fulfil the function of the original one in the protein (formally, any amino acid replacement in a protein is the result of a missense mutation).

Mitosis is the indirect division of a cell that results in the daughter cells acquiring identical genetic information.

Mitochondria are the organelles of the cell where ATP synthesis takes place.

Mitochondrial inheritance **is the** inheritance of traits transmitted through mitochondrial DNA.

Multiple alleles - the presence of more than two alleles of the same locus in a population (or species).

A mosaic is an individual who has cells with different chromosome sets.

Mosaicism is the presence in an individual of cells with two or more variants of chromosome sets.

Mongoloid eye section - lowered inner corners of the eye slits.

Monosomy is the absence of a single chromosome in the karyotype.

Morganida is the distance between two genes with a crossingover frequency of 1% between them.

Congenital morphogenetic variants (synonym: microanomalies of development, signs or stigmas of dysembryogenesis) - developmental abnormalities that go beyond normal variations, but do not disturb the functions of the organism.

Multifactorial diseases (MFDs) are diseases that develop as a result of the interaction of certain combinations of alleles from different loci and specific environmental factors.

Mutagen - a physical, chemical or biological agent that increases the frequency of mutations.

Mutagenesis is the process of causing mutations.

Mutant - an organism carrying a mutant allele.

Frameshift **mutations** are deletions or insertions (insertions) of sections of the DNA molecule whose sizes are not multiples of three bases.

Mutation - a change in hereditary structures (DNA, gene, chromosome, genome).

"Widow's Cape" is a wedge-shaped growth of hair on the forehead.

Hereditary disease is a disease for which the etiological factor is a gene, chromosomal or genomic mutation.

Heritability is part of the total phenotypic variability due to genetic factors.

Nonsense mutations are gene mutations that result in the formation of a terminator codon instead of a sense codon.

Response norm is the range of phenotypic variability for the same genotype under different environmental conditions.

A carrier is an individual who has one copy of the gene that causes the recessive disease and one copy of the normal allele.

Oligodactelia is the absence of one or more fingers.

An oligosonde is a short stretch of DNA, hybridisation with which reveals single base pair substitutions.

Oncogenes are genes that encode proteins that can cause malignant transformation of cells.

Panmixia is the random selection of mating individuals within an entire **population.**

Penetrance is the frequency of manifestation of a phenotype (trait or disease) determined by a dominant allele or recessive allele but in a homozygous state.

Peroxisomal diseases are inherited metabolic diseases caused by impaired biogenesis or function of peroxisomes.

Pleiotropy is the influence of a single gene on the development of two or more phenotypic traits.

The pilonidal fossa is a canal lined with multilayered squamous epithelium that opens in the interjagodic fold at the coccyx.

Polygenic traits are traits caused by many genes, each of which has only the greatest influence on the degree of expression of a given trait.

Polydactyly - an increase in the number of fingers on the hands or feet.

Polymorphism is the presence of several distinctly different phenotypes within a single population.

Restriction fragment length polymorphism (RFLP) is the presence of DNA regions of different lengths after DNA treatment with a particular restrictionase.

A polyploid is a cell (tissue or organism) that has three or more chromosome sets.

Sex chromosomes - chromosomes that determine the sex of an individual (in humans, the Xi U chromosomes).

A population is a group of freely interbreeding individuals of the same species existing in a certain space and time.

Preauricular fistulas are blindly terminated passages whose external opening is located at the base of the ascending part of the auricular curl, anterior to the cochlea or lobe.

Genetic predisposition is a combination of alleles of different loci that predispose to earlier onset of diseases under the influence of environmental factors and their more severe course.

Prenatal diagnosis - diagnosis of inherited diseases or other disorders during intrauterine development.

The proband is the person with whom the collection of ancestry begins.

Prognathia - protrusion of the lower jaw forward compared to the upper jaw.

Progeria is premature aging of the body.

Prognathia - protrusion of the upper jaw forward compared to the lower jaw.

Screening **programmes** - (see screening).

Prophase is the first stage of mitosis.

Pterygium is a wing-shaped fold of skin.

Ptosis is the drooping of the eyelids.

Recombination is the formation of new combinations of genes during meiosis as a result of random cleavage of allele pairs and crossingover.

Recombinant DNA is a DNA molecule "assembled" in a test tube using DNA segments from two different sources.

Restrictases are enzymes that cut DNA at strictly defined sites.

Recessive - a trait or corresponding allele that is only expressed in the homozygous state.

Ribosomes are small intracellular particles composed of rRNA and protein on which polypeptide chains are synthesised.

A pedigree is a chart showing the kinship between members of the same family in a series of generations.

Sandal cleft - the wide space between the first and second toes of the foot.

Familial diseases are diseases seen in several family members in one or more generations.

Sibs are brothers and sisters.

Syndactyly is a complete or partial fusion of the neighbouring fingers of the hand or foot.

Sinophrysis is a conjoined eyebrow.

Screening (synonym; sifting) - the examination of large groups of people to detect any condition (disease or carrier) in order to actively prevent severe forms of disease; the presumptive detection of a previously undiagnosed disease using simple methods that give a quick answer.

Splicing is the process of removing introns and combining exons into a mature mRNA.

A "rocker" foot is a flat-convex plantar surface of the foot with a protruding heel.

Strabismus is **strabismus**.

Gene chaining is the joint transmission of genes (traits).

Telangiectasia - localised excessive dilation of capillaries and small vessels.

Telecanthus - lateral displacement of the inner corners of the ocular slits with normally positioned orbits and eyeballs.

Telomeres are the end sections of chromosomes.

Barr's corpuscles are sex chromatin.

A **tetraploid** is a cell or organism with four sets of chromosomes.

Transgenosis - procedure (or process) of transferring additional foreign genetic information into an organism, cell.

Transcription - reading of hereditary information during gene expression, i.e. synthesis of iRNA on the DNA matrix.

Translocation is the transfer of part of a chromosome, usually to a non-homologous chromosome.

Translation- transfer of hereditary information; synthesis of a protein molecule or translation of the mRNA base sequence into the sequence of amino acids in a polypeptide chain.

Trisomy - the presence of an extra chromosome in the karyotype of a diploid organism; a type of polysomy in which there are three homologous chromosomes (an individual with trisomy is called a trisomic).

Triploid- a cell or organism with three haploid sets of chromosomes.

Short frenulum - attachment of the frenulum in the area of the tip of the tongue or its shortening, resulting in limited mobility of the tongue.

Phenotype - observable traits that are manifested as a result of the action of genes under specific environmental conditions.

Phenocopy - a trait that develops under the influence of environmental factors, but only copies an inherited trait.

Fetoscopy is a procedure that examines the foetus in the uterus using a fibre optic technique.

Fetotherapy - (**fetal** therapy; prenatal therapy)-the treatment of the fetus before birth or immediately after birth.

The filter is the distance from the lower nasal point to the red border of the upper lip.

Phocomelia is the absence or significant underdevelopment of the proximal limbs, causing the normally developed feet and/or hands to appear attached directly to the torso.

Chromatid - two daughter strands of a doubled chromosome joined by a centromere.

Chromosome - nucleoprotein filamentous structures of the cell nucleus containing hereditary information.

A chromosomal mutation (or aberration) is a change in the structure of chromosomes.

Chromosome set - the set of chromosomes in the nucleus of a normal gamete or zygote.

X-linked inheritance **is a** type of inheritance of traits whose genes are localised in the X chromosome.

Centromere - heterochromatin section of the chromosome, which are the attachment site of the "division spindle".

Cyclopia - the presence of a single orbit, located along the midline in the forehead region, containing one or two eyeballs.

An exon is a single fragment of a discontinuous gene that is conserved in mature RNA.

Exophthalmos - displacement of the eyeball forward outside the eye socket; the eye slit is widened.

Expressivity is the degree of phenotypic expression (manifestation) of a genetically determined trait.

Gene expression is the activation of gene transcription, during which mRNA is produced on DNA.

Epicanthus is a vertical skin fold at the inner corner of the eye slit.

Epispadias is an upper urethral cleft, often accompanied by curvature of the penis.

Epistasis is non-allelic dominance.

Euploidy is the presence of complete sets of chromosomes in an individual.

Euchromatin - genetically active regions of chromosomes.

The nucleus organiser is the region of the chromosome containing the genes encoding rRNA.

ANSWERS.

TEST-1.

1. c; karyotype is the number, size and shape of chomosomes in a diploid set.
2. **c;** chromosomes are in equilibrium in the region of the equator.
3. **e;** primordial nucleus fission.
4. b; the acrosome contains an enzyme (hyaluronidase) that helps dissolve the egg shell;
5. **e;** mitotic cell division.

TEST-2. 1. a; 2. c; 3. б; 4. a; 5. д.
TEST-3. 1.c; 2.a; Pros; 4.6;5.c.
TEST-4. 16; 2a; Zs; 4a; 5д.
TEST-5. 1a; 2c; Pros; 4д; 5a.
TEST-6. 1a; 26; Pros; 4д; 5c.
TEST-7. 16; 2a; 3c; 4a; 56.
TEST-8. 16; 26; Zs; 4c; 56.

PROBLEM SOLVING AND ANSWERS

CHALLENGE-1.

1. If you count mitosis, Drosophila has 4 pairs of chromosomes; humans have 23 pairs.

2. a-2n, 4c; b-2n, 2c.

3. 120.

4. in one $6\text{-}10'^{9}$ mg, in two $12\text{-}10'^{9}$ mg; the cause is DNA reduplication.

5. 1) 2n=8; 4A+2XY; 2) 2n=26; 24A+2XX; 3) 2n=80; 78A+ 2XY; 4) 2n=48; 46A+2XX; 5) 2n=46; 44A+2XX.

6. The chromosomal set of mature germ cells of female individuals is 22A+X formula and that of male individuals is 22A+U formula.

7. Chromosome sets of somatic cells and gametes of females and males:
pigs: 38A+XX, 38A+XU; 19A+X, - 19A+U;
grey rat: 40A+XX, 40A+XU; 20A+X, - 20A+U;
rabbit:42A+XX, 42A+XU; 21A+X, - 21A+U.
chimpanzees: 46A+XX, 46A+XU; 23A+X, - 23A+U.

CHALLENGE-2.

1. a). According to the principle of complementarity of nitrogenous bases in the DNA molecule (A - T,C - G), we build the second chain of the molecule:

ААГГЦТЦТАГГТАЦЦАГТ - первая цепочка ДНК
ТТЦЦГАГАТЦЦАТГГТЦА - вторая цепочка ДНК.

б) . According to the principle of complementarity of the nitrogenous bases of DNA and RNA molecules (A - U,C - G), we construct the iRNA chain:

TTC-CGA-GAT-GAT-CCA-TGG-TCA - second DNA strand AAG-GCU-CUA-GGU-ACC-AGU- i-RNA strand

в) . The essence of the code is that the sequence of nucleotides in the iRNA determines the sequence of amino acids in proteins.

<u>AAG-GCU-CUA-CUA-GGU-ACC-AGU-ACC-AGU-</u> I-RNA chain (lys)-(ala)-(leu)-(gly)-(tre)-(ser)-amino acid chain.

2. The nucleotides A and T, G and CD are called ***complementary.*** As a result, in any organism, the number of adenyl nucleotides equals the number of thymidyl nucleotides, and the number of guanyl nucleotides equals the number of cytidyl nucleotides. This regularity was called "E. Chargaff's rule".

Схема: ТТЦЦГАГАТЦЦАТГГТЦА- цепочка ДНК

AAGGTZUCCUAGGUAGGUACCAGU is a molecule of iRNA transcription.

3. Suppose that a protein consists of n monomers - amino acids. Then, its molecular mass will be approximately 110 p. Each amino acid is encoded by three nucleotides; therefore, the DNA chain contains 3 n monomers, and its molecular mass is 300 x 3 p = 900 p. As we see, the molecular mass of a gene (900 p) is approximately 8.2 times higher than the molecular mass (110 p) of the protein it encodes.

4. A protein of 400 monomers is encoded by a sequence of 1200 nucleotides (three nucleotides for each amino acid). The molecular mass of such a coding chain is 300 x 1200=360000. A nucleic acid molecule with a molecular mass of 107 can contain approximately 28 genes (107 : 3.6 x 105), i.e. this is the number of different proteins that can be encoded in it.

5. In the conditions of the problem, code triplets of all amino acids excreted in the urine of a patient with cystinuria are given. Using the code table, we can find out which amino acids are present in the urine of a sick person: serine, cysteine, alanine, glycine, glutamine, arginine, lysine. Amino acids excreted in a healthy person are specified in the task. If we exclude them from the list, we will find out the answer to the question posed in point 1: cysteine, glutamine, arginine, lysine.

CHALLENGE-3.

1. (a)

sign	Gene	Genotype
Normal hearing	*B*	*BB, BB*
Deaf-mute	*B*	*bb*

P ♀ *Bb* x ♂ *Bb*

G *B* *b* *B* *b*

F_1 *BB*, *Bb*, *Bb*, *bb*

Answer: The probability of having a healthy baby is 75%, while the probability of having a sick baby is 25%.

(б)

P ♀ *bb* x ♂ *B_*

G *b* *B* –

F_1 *bb* *B*-

Answer: Since deaf-mute is a recessive trait, the mother's genotype will be *bb*. The father's genotype can be *BB* or *Bb* - in both cases it will be healthy. But the child was born sick, hence, he got one recessive gene from the mother, and the second one should have been given by the father. So the father's genotype *is Bb.*

2. (a) Homozygotes, according to the formula N = 2n , form one type of gamete (20 = 1):

P aabb

G *ab*

б) Heterozygotes for one trait give two types of gametes (21 =2): P AABB G *AB AB aB*

в) Heterozygotes for two traits give four types of gametes (22 = 4): P AaBb G *AB aB aB Ab ab ab*

г) Homozygotes give one type of gamete (20 =1): RAABSS

G *ABC*

д) Heterozygotes for one trait give two types of gametes (21 =2): RAABSS

G *Abc, abc*

e) Hetcrozygotes for three traits give rise to eight types of gametes (23): R AABBCs

G *ABC, aBC, abc, abc, abe, abc, abe, abc, abc.* **3.**

Given:

B, clubfoot; b, normal foot structure; D, normal carbohydrate metabolism; d, diabetes mellitus; $, normal foot structure, normal carbohydrate metabolism;

$ is a slash with normal carbohydrate metabolism;

Fl: 1) only the squint;

2) diabetes only

This task is for dihybrid crossbreeding. Two traits are analysed - foot structure and type of carbohydrate metabolism. Foot structure is represented by two alternative traits. The condition explicitly states which of these traits are dominant and which are recessive. Therefore, it is easy to enter the gene designations and make a brief note of the problem condition.

Solution:

The problem condition does not explicitly say what ge-no-types the parents and children have. Therefore, when writing down the problem, we denote the places of alleles of genes in the genotypes of both parents and children by dots:

P: ♂.... x ♀....

Gametes:

F1: №1....; №2....

At the first stage of solving this problem, it is necessary to fully restore the genotypes of parents and children. This can be done partially using the information from the problem condition. It says that the mother has a normal foot structure and normal carbohydrate metabolism.

Normal foot structure is a recessive trait, so for it to manifest in the phenotype a woman must have two recessive alleles of the **B (bb)** gene.

Fi: - a leering diabetic?

Knowing that she still has normal carbohydrate metabolism, it is natural to assume the presence of at least one dominant **D** allele **(D_)** in her genotype. It is not yet known whether the mother is homozygous or heterozygous for this trait, so the second allele is still denoted by a dot.

The father has normal carbohydrate metabolism and therefore at least one dominant allele of the D gene (D_) and clubfoot (since it is not known whether he is hetero-zygous or homozygous for this trait, we can only record B_).

Similarly, let's reconstruct the genotypes of the children: the first child has only clubfoot, therefore, we can say that he has at least one dominant gene from each pair of traits (B.D.). The second suffers only from diabetes. For the child to have diabetes, he must possess two recessive alleles of the D gene (dd), and for him to phenotypically have a normal structure - feet, he must have two recessive alleles of the (B) gene - (bb). Thus, the second child is digomozygous for recessive traits. The record of the solution of the problem at this stage has the following form:

Solution:

P: ♂ B _ D_ x ♀ bbD _

Gametes:

Fl:#1B_D_; #2 bbdd

Now we can fully restore the genotypes of the parents using the following reasoning: at fertilisation, the zygote receives one homologous chromosome from the mother's egg and the second one from the father's sperm. Hence, one gamete with recessive alleles (bd) is derived from the mother and the second gamete with the same allele is derived from the father. So both mother and father must have both recessive alleles (b) and (d) in their genotype. Thus, the fully reconstructed genotype of the parents is as follows:

P: ♂ BbDd x ♀ bbDd

Now we have everything we need to answer the main question of the problem. However, this requires writing out all types of gametes formed by both father and mother. The analysis shows that the father gives 4 types of gametes, and the mother - 2 types.

P: ♂ **BbDd** x ♀ **bbDd**

gametes: BD; Bd, bD; bd;

bD; bd;

To determine the probable genotypes of the offspring, let us make a Pennett lattice. The father's gametes, for example, will be written in the upper horizontal line, and the mother's gametes in the left vertical line. In the places of intersection write down the genotypes of the offspring.

♂♀	BD	Bd	bd	bd
bD	BbDD	BbDd	bbDD	bbDd
bd	BbDd	Bbdd	bbDd	bbdd

It can be seen that there is only I variant of children with the desired phenotype. Consequently, the probability of giving birth to a diabetic child (with both anomalies) in this couple is:

Splitting by genotype:

IBbDD : 2BbDd : 2bbDd : IBbdd : IbbDD : 1bbdd

Phenotype splitting:

3 :	**3 :**	**1**	**1**
clubfoot, normal carbohydrate metabolism	*normal foot, normal carbohydrate metabolism*	*clubfoot, diabetes*	*normal foot, diabetes* **1** *normal foot, diabetes*

R: 3+3+1+1+1 = 8 out of eight is one squint. If you count 8 - 100% 1- 12.5%

When solving problems of this type, it should be borne in mind that the calculation of the probability of having children does not take into account the fact that a given parental couple already has children.

Answer: the probability of having children with both anomalies is 12.5%.

4. This problem requires analysis of one pair of traits, familial hypercholesterolemia. This trait is autosomal dominant. Since the parents have only high cholesterol content in the blood, they are heterozygotes. A brief note of the problem condition will look as follows:

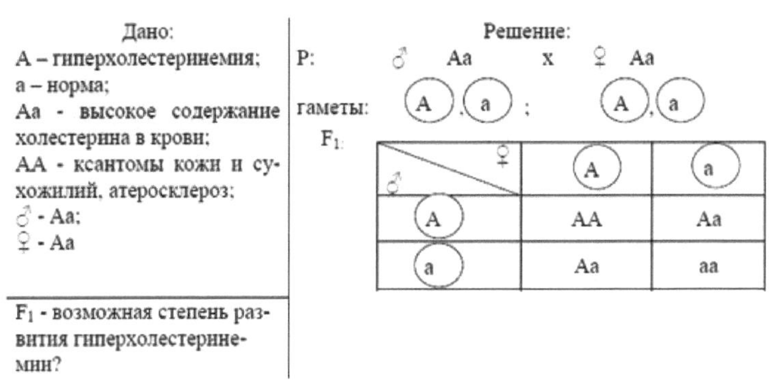

Расщепление в F_1 по генотипу и фенотипу:

1АА	:	2Аа	:	1аа
ксантомы кожи и сухожилий, атеросклероз		высокое содержание холестерина в крови		норма

Given:

A - hypercholesterolaemia: a - normal;

Aa - high cholesterol in the blood;

AA - xanthomas of the skin and tendons. atherosclerosis; d-Aa;

? - Aah! Aah!

Fi - possible degree of hypercholesterolemia myia?

Stratification in F_t by genotype and phenotype} :[7]

1AA : 2AA : laa

skin xanthomas

"the norm.

n tendonitis, atherosclerosis blood cholesterol

Sometimes alleles that, in the heterozygous state, determine the development of a trait, in the homozygous state are lethal to the organism. Such alleles are called lethal alleles. For example, in humans, the dominant brachydactyly mutation in the heterozygous state manifests itself in the form of shortened fingers. However, in the homozygous state, this gene leads to death in the early stages of development, due to the resulting skeletal deformities incompatible with life. When analysing the lethal manifestation of the trait, the Mendelian cleavage formula becomes 2:1.

6. The problem condition gives direct clear indications about the genotypes of the parents. Therefore, we can guess that the mother's genotype is I^A i and the father's genotype is I I^{AB} . Let's make a multiple notation of the condition:

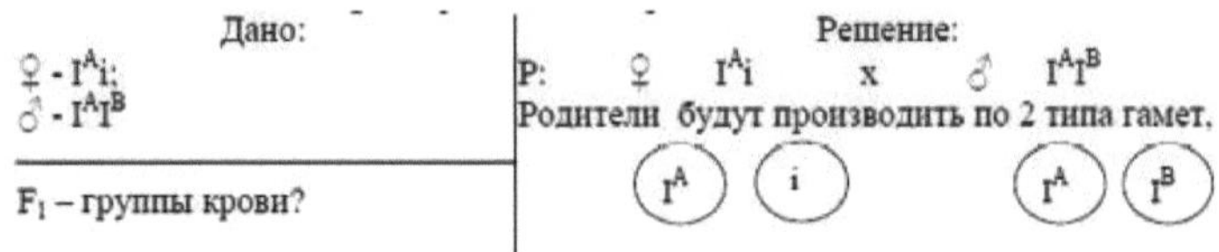
Дано:
♀ - I^Ai;
♂ - I^AI^B

F_1 – группы крови?

Решение:
P: ♀ I^Ai x ♂ I^AI^B
Родители будут производить по 2 типа гамет.
I^A i I^A I^B

Для выявления сочетания генов в F_1 составим решетку Пеннета:

F_1:

♀ \ ♂	I^A	I^B
I^A	I^AI^A	I^AI^B
i	I^Ai	I^Bi

Генотип: 1 I^AI^A : 1 I^Ai : 1 I^AI^B : 1 I^Bi
Фенотип: II(A) II(A) IV(AB) III(B)

To identify the combination of genes in Fi, we make a Pennett lattice:
Genotype: 1 I I^{AA} : 1 I^A i: 1 I I^{AB} : 1 I i^B
Phenotpp: 11(A) 11(A) 11(A) IV(AB) 111(B)

CHALLENGE-4.

1. Aneuploidy is trisomy on the sex chromosomes. Chromosome misalignment during meiosis during ovogenesis or spermatogenesis:

a) an egg with two X chromosomes and a sperm containing a Y chromosome fuse;

б) an egg with an X chromosome and a sperm with X and Y chromosomes fuse. Such men are infertile (Klinefelter syndrome).

2. This chromosomal mutation may involve abnormalities of meiosis during spermatogenesis. Four variants of spermatozoa can be formed:

1. 23 chromosomes, chromosome 21 is free;
2. 23 chromosomes, but chromosome 21 is translocated;
3. 24 chromosomes at the expense of two chromosomes 21, free and translocated;
4. 22 chromosomes, chromosome 21 is missing.

Thus, there is a high probability of having children with Down's disease.

3. formalise the problem condition in the form of a table:

sign	Gene	Genotype	Gene localisation
Rhesus-positive blood	*D*	*D-*	one autosome:
Ellpptozptoz	*E1*	*E1-*	
Rhesus-negative blood	*d*	*dd*	distance *D* - *E1* = *3* morganpdas
The normal shape of red blood cells	*el*	*elel*	

1). We determine the genotype of the woman by the phenotype of her parents - she is heterozygous for the elliptocytosis genes and the presence of the Rh factor:

$$\frac{dEl}{Del}$$

2). We determine the genotype of the husband - he is homozygous for recessive alleles d and el:

$$\frac{del}{del}$$

3) . Write down the pattern of the marriage.

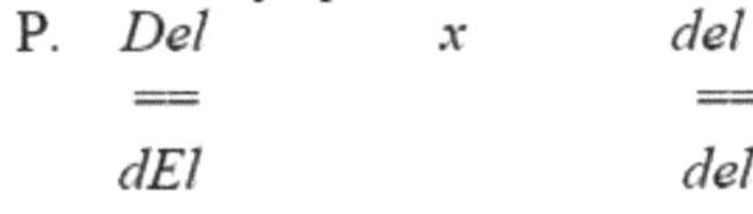

P. $\frac{Del}{dEl}$ x $\frac{del}{del}$

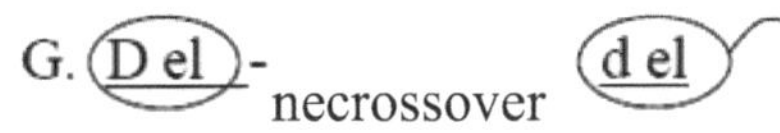

G. D el - necrossover d el

d El - necrossover

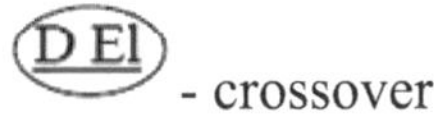

D El - crossover

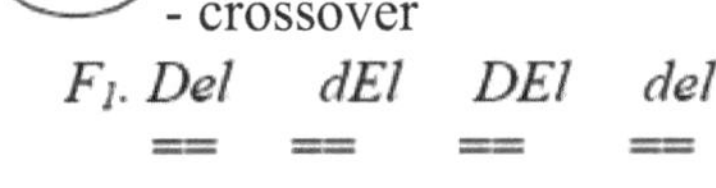

d el - crossover

F_1. $\frac{Del}{del}$ $\frac{dEl}{del}$ $\frac{DEl}{del}$ $\frac{del}{del}$

4) We calculate the percentage of crossover and necrossover gametes. Cross-over gametes - 3% (1.5% each), as the distance between genes is 3 morganids, necrossover gametes - 97% (48.5% each).

5) . Each gamete can receive only one of the homologous chromosomes. The probability of formation in a woman of gametes with genes Del - 48,5%, dEl - 48,5%, DEl - 1,5%, del - 1,5%. The husband has gametes of the same type - del.

6) . We determine the probability of giving birth to children with the combinations of traits specified in the problem condition. It depends on the

probability of fusion of gametes of different types: a) 48.5%; b) 1.5%; c) 48.5%; d) 1.5%.

4. Phenocopy. The rubella virus has prevented the genes responsible for the development of the hearing organ from realising their information. Deafness here is a non-hereditary trait, so the probability of a deaf child being born again is 0 unless the mother has a recurrence during pregnancy. The son's wife has hereditary deafness, she is homozygous for the deafness gene, but the children will have normal hearing because they receive the dominant gene for normal hearing from their father; they will be heterozygous carriers of the deafness gene.

5. The disease is associated, firstly, with mutational variability (generative mutation in one of Edik's ancestors), which resulted in the phenylketonuria gene in this family. Secondly, with combinative variability, due to which this gene became homozygous. Edik's recovery is due to modification variability. Edik's genotype did not change, but appropriate external influences normalised his phenotype.

CHALLENGE-5.

1. On the basis of anamnesis data build a family tree.

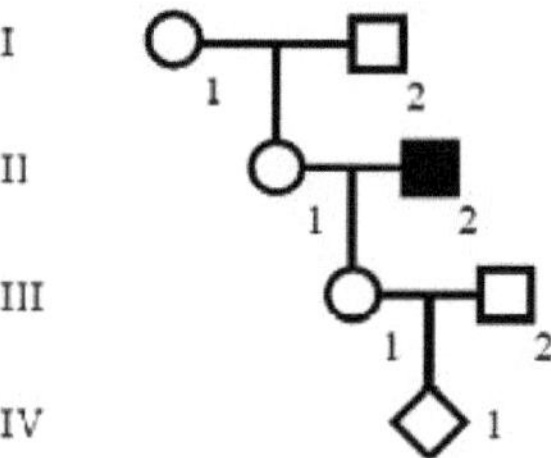

Then we draw up the problem condition in the form of a table and write down the genetic scheme of marriage:

A woman who is going to have a child is heterozygous for the ichthyosis gene. The probability of giving birth to a sick child in marriage with a healthy man is 25% of all children, 50% if a boy is born and 0% if a girl. Chorionbiopsy (8-12 weeks of pregnancy) and amniocentesis (15-17 weeks of pregnancy) are indicated to clarify the possibility of giving birth to a sick child. The methods allow to determine the presence of X-sex chromatin in fetal cells to establish the sex.

sign	Gene	G enotnp
Ichthyosis	y^7	XX^I, XY

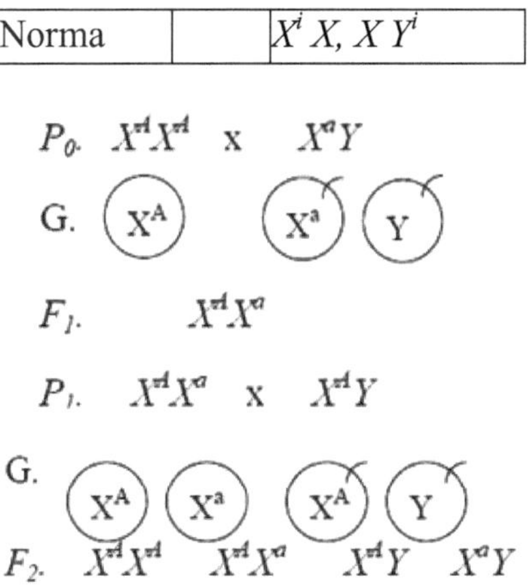

Norma		$X^i X, X Y^i$

If the sex of the future child is found to be male (genetic risk of 50%), the geneticist must explain the severity of the medical consequences of the disease and recommend an induced termination of pregnancy. If the foetus is found to be female, the risk of having a sick child is 0%. The woman who is going to have a child is heterozygous for the ichthyosis gene. The probability of having a sick child in a marriage with a healthy man is 25% of all children, 50% if a boy is born, and 0% if a girl.

2. Heterozygous parents Aa and Aa marry. Phenotypically they are healthy. When heterozygous parents marry, the genotypes of the children are probable:

sign	Gene	G enotpp
Norma	*A*	*AA, Aa*
Phenylketonuria (disease)	*a*	*aah*

AA - 25 per cent, Aa - 50 per cent, Aa - 25 per cent.

Hence, the probability of having healthy children is 75% and the probability of having children with phenylketonuria is 25%.

3. formalise the problem condition in the form of a table:

sign	Gene	Genotype
Blood type I (0)	I^0	I^0I^0
Blood type II (A)	I^A	I^AI^A, I^AI^0
Blood type III (B)	I^B	I^BI^B, I^BI^0
IV (AB) blood group	I^A *u* I^B	I^AI^B
Secretors	*S*, I^A, I^B	S- I^A I, S- I^B I

Nonsecretors	*s* *S u I⁰*	*ss* *S-I⁰I⁰*

P. I^BIss x I^AIS-

F1. I^AI^Bss I⁰I⁰ S S-

Since the second child has blood group I (genotype I I^{00}), each of the parents must have gene 10 in their genotype, so they are heterozygous for blood group (they have genotypes I I^{B0} and 1^{A} I°). Since the first child does not have antigens A and B in his saliva, he has two recessive ss genes in his genotype, which he got from each of his parents.

B0 A0

Thus, it is not possible to determine the genotype of the second child by the secretor-nonsecretor gene.

4. formalise the problem condition in the form of a table:

attribute	**Gene**	**Genotype**
Brown eyes	*A*	*A-*
Blue eyes	*A*	*Aa*
Dark hair colour	*B*	*B-*
Light hair colour	*B*	*VY*

Each parent has one dominant trait and one recessive trait, so their genotypes are as follows:

father *is aaB-,* mother *is aaB-.*

Since their four children are different, it means that their phenotypes and genotypes are so:

- The first child is a brown-eyed, dark-haired (*A-B-*);
- the second child is a brown-eyed, blonde-haired (*A-ЪЪ*);
- The third child is a blue-eyed, dark-haired (*aaB-*);
- The fourth child is a blue-eyed, blonde-haired (*aabb*).

Knowing the genotype of the fourth child, it is possible to establish the genotypes of the parents, since each of them must pass two recessive genes to this child: *aЪ*.

Thus, the father's genotype is *AaBb and the* mother's genotype is *Aabb.*

5. (A) According to the conditions of the problem, a healthy woman, whose brother has haemophilia, married a healthy man. During biochemical analysis of blood coagulation factors, it is found that the disease is caused by deficiency of Christmas factor. The diagnosis was haemophilia *B*. The disease is inherited as a sex-linked recessive trait. Pedigree analysis confirmed this finding and showed that the mother of the woman seeking advice was heterozygous. The penetrance of haemophilia is 100%. In determining the probability of having a sick child, we first note that the counselled woman's genotype could be either X X^{BB} , or X X^{Bb} . Since her mother is heterozygous X X^{Bb} , and her father's genotype is X^{B} Y , the probability that she is homozygous is 1/2, as is the probability that she is heterozygous. The probability of a heterozygous woman having a sick child when married to a normal man is 1/4. Therefore, the probability that the child from this marriage will have haemophilia is

1/2 x 1/4=1/8 (12,5%).

In counselling this case, the physician should keep the following circumstances in mind:

Firstly, if with positive advice from a counsellor, a family wants to have two children, the probability that one of them will be sick is 1/8+1/8=1/4.

Secondly, the probability of having a heterozygous carrier is 1/8 for one child in a family and 1/4 for two.

The probability of the haemophilia gene being passed on to offspring (patients + carriers) is 1/4 if there is one child in the family. If a family has two children, the probability that one of them will be either sick or a carrier is 50%.

CHALLENGE-6.

1. The girls will all have enamel hypoplasia, and among the boys the cleavage is 1:1 (there is a 25% chance of having a son with normal teeth).

2. The girls will be normal vision, but one of them is a carrier of colour blindness. Boys are 50 per cent normal vision, 50 per cent girls.

3. Since the son has both anomalies, hence the mother was diheterozygous and the father heterozygous for the second pair of genes. The probability of being born with two anomalies is 1/16 - 6.25%.

4. 1) 47,XX,13+; 2) 47,XHU,18+ ;3) 47, XHU ,21+; 4) 47,XHU; 5) 45,X.

5) 1) female karyotype, 46 chromosomes, elongated short arm of the first chromosome;

6) male karyotype, deletion of the long arm of chromosome 14;

7) female karyotype, 46 chromosomes with an elongated short arm of chromosome 14;

8) female karyotype, 46 chromosomes, deletion of chromosome 1 (in the first segment, second region of the long arm of chromosome 21);

9) male karyotype, 45 autosomal chromosomes long arm translocation from chromosome 14 to chromosome 21 (see Appendices No. 3).

10) female karyotype, 46 chromosomes, ring chromosome 18.

CHALLENGE-7.

1. For a small population, the mathematical expression of the Hardy-Weinberg law cannot be applied, so it is not possible to calculate gene frequencies.

2. Formalise the problem condition in the form of a table:

sign	Gene	Genotype
Disease Tay-Sachs	*A*	*Aah*
Norma	*A*	*A-*

We make a mathematical notation of the Hardy-Weinberg law p + q = 1, p2 + 2pq + q2 = 1.

p - frequency of occurrence of the A gene;

q is the frequency of occurrence of gene a;

p2 - frequency of occurrence of dominant homozygotes (AA);

2pq is the frequency of occurrence of heterozygotes (Aa);

q2 - frequency of recessive homozygotes (aa).

From the problem condition, according to the Hardy-Weinberg formula, we know the frequency of occurrence of sick children (aa), i.e. q2 = 1/5000. The gene causing this disease will be passed to the next generation only from heterozygous parents, so it is necessary to find the frequency of occurrence of heterozygotes (Aa), i.e. 2pq.

q = 1/71, p =1-q = 70/71, 2pq = 0.028.

We determine the concentration of the gene in the next generation. It will be in 50% of gametes in heterozygotes, its concentration in the gene pool is about 0.014. The probability of giving birth to sick children q2 = 0.000196, or 0.98 per 5000 population. Thus, the concentration of the pathological gene and the frequency of this disease in the next generation of this population will not practically change (there is a slight decrease).

3. formalise the problem condition in the form of a table:

sign	Gene	Genotype
Norma	*a*	*Aah*
Hip dislocation	*A*	*A-*

Thus, from the problem condition, according to the Hardy-Weinberg formula, we know the frequency of occurrence of genotypes AA and Aa, i.e. *p2+2pq*. It is necessary to find the frequency of occurrence of genotype Aa, i.e. *q2*.

From the formula *p2+ 2pq + q2=1* it is clear that the number of individuals homozygous for the recessive gene *(aa) q2=l-(p2+2pq)*. However, the number of diseased individuals given in the problem (6: 10,000) does not represent p2 + 2pq, but only 25 per cent of the carriers of gene A, while the true number of people carrying the gene is four times more, i.e. 24 : 10,000. Hence, *p2 + 2pq* =24:10,000. Then q2 (the number of individuals homozygous for the recessive gene) is 9976: 10 000.

4. The trait does not occur in every generation. This rules out the dominant type of inheritance. Since the trait occurs in both males and females, this rules out hollandric type of inheritance. To rule out the sex-linked recessive type of inheritance, it is necessary to consider the III-3 and III-4 mating pattern (the trait does not occur in males and females). In this case if to assume that genotype of the man X^A Y, and genotype of the woman X^A X^a , they cannot have a daughter with this trait (X^a X^a), and in the given pedigree there is a daughter with this trait - IV-2. Taking into account the occurrence of the trait equally in both men and women and the case of close marriage, we can conclude that in this pedigree there is an autosomal recessive type of inheritance.

5. Use Holzinger's formula to calculate the inheritance coefficient:

$$H = \frac{\text{КМБ\%} - \text{КДБ\%}}{100\% - \text{КДБ\%}}$$

$$H = \frac{80\% - 30\%}{100\% - 30\%} = 0{,}71$$

Since the inheritability coefficient is 0.71, genotype plays a major role in the formation of the trait.

CHALLENGE-8.

1. The trait does not occur in every generation. This rules out dominant inheritance. Since the trait occurs in both males and females, this rules out hollandric inheritance. To exclude the sex-linked recessive type of inheritance, it is necessary to consider the marriage pattern III-3 and III-4 (the trait does not occur in males and females). In this case, if we assume that the genotype of the man is XAY and the genotype of the woman is XAHa, they cannot have a daughter with this trait (XAHa), and in this pedigree there is a daughter with this trait - IV-2. Taking into account the occurrence of the trait equally in both males and females and the case of close marriage, we can conclude that in this pedigree there is an autosomal recessive type of inheritance.

2. X-linked recessive type of inheritance.

3. X-linked dominant type of inheritance.

4. The presence of haemophilia in the son indicates that his mother (the female counsellor) has the haemophilia gene. The father also has the haemophilia gene. Therefore, there is a high probability (50%) of haemophilia not only in the son but also in the daughter who may be homozygous for the gene. In both cases there are equal indications for termination of pregnancy, but given the modern techniques of molecular genetic methods, it is possible to carry out amniocentesis, find in the amniotic fluid of the fetus cells and by gene fingerprinting to detect the presence or absence of the pathological gene in the genotype. If it is absent, the pregnancy should be maintained.

5. c) subluxation of the lens, heart defects, tall stature, long thin fingers, funnel-shaped depression of the sternum;

REFERENCE LIST

1. A.Y.Asanov, N.S.Demikova, S.A.Morozov, Edited by A.Y.Asanov. "Fundamentals of genetics and hereditary developmental disorders in children" textbook for students. Higher Pedagogical Educational Institutions/M: Publishing Centre "Academy", 2003.
2. P.R.Olimkhodjaeva, D.R.Inogamova. "Medical genetics". - T., Ibn Sino, 2002.
3. D.R. Inogamova. "Collection of didactic materials and tasks on medical genetics". - T., Turon-Ikbol, 2005.
4. D.R. Inogamova. "Medical genetics". - T, Chulpan, 2009.
5. V.S.Baranov, E.V.Baranova, T.E.Ivashchenko, M.V.Aseev. "The human genome and 'predisposition' genes". "Introduction to Predictive Medicine". - SPb.: Intermedica, 2000.
6. N.P. Bochkov. "Clinical Genetics". - Moscow: Medicine, 1997.
7. E.T.Lilin, E.A.Bogomazov, P.B.Hoffman-Kadoshnikov. "Genetics for physicians". - Moscow, Medicine, 1990.
8. A.A.Kamensky, A.I.Kim, L.L.Velikanov, O.D.Lopatina, S.A.Balandin et al. "Biology". - M., Slovo, 2001.
9. D.K.Belyaev, G.M.Dymshits. "General biology". - M., Prosveshchenie, 2001.
10. F. Vogel, A. Motulski. "Human genetics." In 3 vol. -M., Mir, 1989.
11. P. Harper. "Practical medical and genetic counselling". - M., Medicine, 1984.

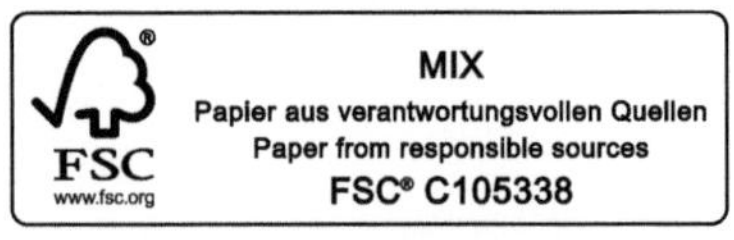

Printed by Books on Demand GmbH, Norderstedt / Germany